Naturopathic Reiki II

The Essentials of Therapy

K. Akua Gray
Curriculum Development Coordinator
A Life Of Peace Wellness Education Institute, Inc.
Houston, TX

BJK Publishing and Distribution, LLC
Houston, TX
2017

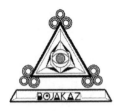

Bojakaz Management
P O Box 921
Missouri City, Texas 77459

This publication was designed to provide accurate and au-
thoritative information in regard to the subject matters
covered. It is sold with the intention to educate, inform,
and empower readers to make their own decisions on
health, life, and well-being. If you have concerns about
your physical, mental, or spiritual condition consult the
appropriate professional.

Cover Design: K. Akua Gray and Cover Fresh Design
Cover Photo: G. Chenu Gray

Printed in the United States of America
ISBN 10: 0-9904089-7-3
ISBN-13: 978-0-9904089-7-0

To the light of love that awakens every healer
to fulfill their divine purpose

Also by K. Akua Gray

Naturopathic Reiki I: Opening the Way

☥

Naturopathic Reiki III: The Power of the Master

☥

Natural Health and Wellness: The Consultant Manual

☥

Holistic Sexuality: A Practical Guide to Sexual Healing

☥

Today: Wellness Manifestations

☥

Veggie Delights: Holistic Health Recipes,
Eating Live for Maximum Nutrition and Wellness

☥

Akwaaba!: Dr. Akua's Ghanaian Vegan Cuisine

Table of Contents

Foreword

Having owned a complementary and alternative practice that provides products and services incorporating various holistic modalities for seven years, it is an honor to write about the significance of Naturopathic Reiki II: The Essentials of Therapy. Reiki is one of the modalities I've used extensively for over 6 years as a certified Reiki Master Teacher and Healing Touch Practitioner Student. My personal holistic health and wellness journey started in 1993, but began to blossom into a business only after becoming acquainted with Dr. Akua Gray in 2010. She has practiced and taught a plethora of natural health and wellness modalities while emphasizing the importance of healing yourself, family and community. Dr. Gray uses her educational background in developing holistic therapy curriculums by identifying the most salient points of a subject and making it understandable and relevant to your daily life. Her proficient skills and ability to successfully deliver professional courses further demonstrates her vast knowledge in natural health and wellness services and modalities.

In my Reiki experience, I've come to a knowing that this therapy is healing for both the client and the therapist. One of my experiences was working with an elderly female client whom suffered with insomnia, incontinence, severe osteoarthritis, strong Christian beliefs, unmanageable high blood pressure, high cholesterol, and rigid right and wrong behavioral expectations. She was a little apprehensive at first, but decided it wouldn't hurt if she, "tried it this one time." After receiving an hour of Reiki she slept for over 2 hours and upon waking she was able to walk without pain, felt rested, blood pressure lowered, less argumentative and experienced an open and optimistic view of life. She understood it wasn't a cure and that it was temporary without changing her lifestyle, however in her view it was well worth a moment of peace. She continued to request Reiki services until her spiritual realm transition. This experience helped me to actually see instant results of administered Reiki for myself and it removed any doubts about the practice while building confidence and instilling a drive to practice and learn more. Practicing Reiki regularly continues to reveal new metaphysical gifts and strengthens realized ones. This therpy continuously evolves as you consistently apply the principles in your life.

Through my training experience and many of my students I've recognized that oft time new students get so excited after their initial training that there's an immediate desire to have metaphysical experiences and when progress seems slow, frustration develops. That said, I've also noticed an increased quest for more knowledge and certifications without application of principles already learned. The strength about Dr. Gray's teaching style is that she shares techniques to enhance your experience through suggested activities to be completed in a particular timeframe to further prepare your mind, body and spirit for continued growth in this powerful enlightening journey.

Reiki is the most known and widely used form of energy medicine performed in the U.S.A. today. The Usui System of Reiki originated in Japan by Dr. Mikao Usui and was introduced to the West by Mrs. Hawayo Takata. After years of practicing Usui Reiki Dr. Gray acknowledges that over time at an energetic level, portals of creativity were opened and guided her development of Naturopathic Reiki. She discusses new techniques to specifically assist naturopathic therapist while maintaining the original Usui principles in this book.

Reiki reminds me of the ancient practice of "laying on of hands". The power of touch to heal has been practiced and in some instances still practiced in Greek mythology, Christianity, Judaism, Shamanism and other ancient traditional healers. I mention this because so many of us initially are apprehensive about things we know little about or have social conditioning that fosters a negative image.

Many cultures and religions utilize the "laying on of hands" to symbolically demonstrate the receiving of the Holy Spirit or a spiritual exchange for healing. To me Reiki is the "laying on of hands" with the science of physiology applied to focus specific intent to the aura, body temple and mental areas of our being. That said, the practitioner's inner power paves the way to dive deeper to uncover one's mental, physical and spiritual blockages and stagnations. This allows the Reiki therapist to target specific organs and other areas of the body to help facilitate the client's self-healing.

Pointing out a great deal about how his book enhances a therapist's skills and service portfolio, I feel there would be a disservice not to share the value this modality has for a layperson. Dis-eases and discomfort from aliments like Post Traumatic Stress Disorder (PTSD), Post Traumatic Slave Syndrome, depression, bipolar disorder, joint pain, high blood pressure, migraine headaches, post-partum and many others can be improved through the use of the techniques in this book. You and your family could potentially reduce your doctor visits and medications resulting in money saved, reduced medical complications and jump start self-healing. I am by no means stating this is a cure nor am I suggesting you start the practice without talking to your licensed healthcare provider, however studies by The Center of Reiki Research along with Healing Touch Professional Association and experience has shown positive progress.

Naturopathic Reiki II: The Essentials of Therapy builds on the knowledge learned in Naturopathic Reiki I and Usui Reiki I. This book is a text and reference manual that has been built to foster increased Reiki skills with new tools and techniques. Dr. Akua Gray shares therapist preparation, self-practice recommendations, expands symbols utilized by the addition of Ancient African symbols and the application of crystal therapy to further enhance the healing skills of the naturopathic therapist.

D'or Nelson
Naturopathic Therapist
Usui Reiki Master Teacher
Life Force Counselor

Introduction

Moving forward with your Reiki training can take many different paths. Over the past forty years quite a few systems of Reiki have developed from several unique perspectives, however, all of them have the foundation of Reiki as it was taught in Usui Shiki Ryoho. The Reiki Principles, the standard hand positions, and the intention that Reiki is to be used for the greater good of humanity is well established. When something is as good as Reiki on an energy level it opens portals of creativity for those who take this healing and spiritual art seriously. One such portal of creativity has opened up recently in the realm of naturopathy and has brought forth an expansion of knowledge in the world of Reiki that is specifically designed to assist naturopathic therapists with an exclusive version of this energy work that will take their service of health and wellness to great heights.

Naturopathic Reiki is an expansive health therapy that raises the vibration of the spirit, the mind, the emotions and the physical body. As we are aware, Source has no limitations and is deemed immeasurable with the sun being a prime example to the vastness of energy that we experience daily. I personally find it quite enriching to know that Reiki as a healing art is not stuck in ridged protocols but instead has taken on a history of uniqueness with accountability to its origins.

Naturopathic Reiki II is in alignment with the Shinpi Den (*the secrets/mystery* teachings) where intermediate students are introduced to the Reiki Symbols, advance hand placements for specific conditions, healing programs, techniques for remote healing and the complete concepts for professional therapy. This training manual has evolved with over ten years of nurturing and attuning more than two hundred students of Reiki. The majority of the students began at the level of first degree, which is primarily used for personal health. However, there have been many who have gone on to the second degree to learn about the professional therapist aspect of Reiki and the greater spiritual enrichments that can be found at this level. Some have even broadened their horizons to become Naturopathic Reiki Master Teachers and are now working throughout the communities of the United States of America, Canada, Israel, Ghana, Kenya, Nigeria, Senegal, The United Kingdom, Switzerland, The Bahamas, and Japan.

It is our greatest intention to provide a work of enlightenment for seekers who are destined for this path. Like many trailblazers in Reiki before me who have set the tone to develop and expand new ideas in Reiki, I offer this unique expansion as a guide to develop naturopathic therapists of Reiki who do the work of balancing themselves physically, mentally, emotionally and spiritually first and then take the confidence of their own healing with them as they expand the globe healing the world.

Chapter 1

seeks to help bring people to wholeness

Reiki II
The Naturopathic Perspective

The second degree of Naturopathic Reiki training focuses on the use of specific energy. As light workers who have begun the journey of Reiki with self-healing at the first degree, you are now ready to expand into the world of health care using Reiki for others. There are four areas of focus as outlined in _Naturopathic Reiki I: Opening the Way_, that serve as the foundation to maximizing the effects of Reiki and its ability to nurture purpose in every individual.

Physical imbalances such as pain, disease, and any other health issue reduces the vibration of a person and blocks their ability to radiate at high energy levels.

Physical solutions come through the advanced modalities of Naturopathic Reiki that we will learn about in this book as well as by using other physical solutions that have been tested, lived and experienced with positive outcomes.

Mental imbalances such as judgmental behavior, prejudice, negative thinking, and religious fanaticism deprives a person of peace of mind and fuels emotional dysfunctionality. Many ailments that people suffer from take place in the mind.

Mental solutions are engrained in the use of the Reiki symbols that are a primary goal of mastery at the second degree. To give power to the mind to seek balance is the first step. The second step is to encourage the mind to develop consistent efforts and rituals for change. Third is to fortify the mind with peace knowledge that promotes ways of living that makes turning back to old ways impossible.

Emotions are barriers
to spiritual ascension

Emotional imbalances such as fear, sadness, anger, and any other emotional crutch, blocks the ability to be spiritually complete and live life well. Emotional immaturity that openly display negative emotions are usually the primary means of dysfunctional behavior.

Emotional solutions are also engrained in the use of the Reiki symbols with an emphasis on aligning the energy portals of the body to feel peace. The goal is to make feeling of peace a way of life.

Spiritual imbalances are reflected in all of the above. When the spirit is completely nurtured and receptive to actions of purpose learning a person has achieved the ultimate goal of balance.

Spiritual solutions are grounded in the truth that Reiki is effective on every unseen level. Spirit has no boundaries of space, time or distance and the quietness that assures its presence is available to the therapist and the client.

As a Naturopathic Reiki II therapist one of the goals is to relax psychological tensions with the advanced work of releasing physical, mental, emotional and spiritual energy blocks. You will learn to be a vibrant conduit for universal power.

As a conductor for your clients on the Naturopathic Reiki II level, your ability to create healthcare plans that address the physical, mental, emotional and spiritual aspects of your clients gives you a greater purpose in using Reiki for healing. Assessment is the foundation of the seriousness of your work with your clients. During your initial consultation before therapy, you will inquire about the most important things that may be of a pressing nature with your clients in four

We are putting together wellness therapy programs

simple questions.

1. Are there any physical issues you would like for us to work on?
2. Are there any mental blocks that are stopping you from making the most of everyday?
3. Are you carrying around any emotional baggage? — *ask about relationships*
4. Are you spiritually satisfied with every aspect of your life?

You can choose to speak in detail with your clients about their answers or you can have them give you a short list which lets you know immediately where energy blockages are apparent. We will expand on this in the upcoming chapter on Reiki Chakra Therapy.

Naturopathic Reiki II teaches specific health therapy techniques and programs that can induce new perspectives on life by coming face to face with what is keeping a person from accessing their higher self. The higher self is a place of tranquil action that everyone must access in order to change. In these health therapies, we are taught to use natural tools such as crystals and the elements as physical reminders of what source has provided. Sometimes your clients are being taught this for the first time, and for others you will be opening the portals for them to remember their divine power.

You are the vessel through which divine energy is working. Honor yourself and the power within that brought you to this healing art. The world is in need of more spiritual health care providers. Be who you were created to be.

Chapter 1 Summary

The second degree of Reiki must be full circle in the health process. It has been noted in every healing profession that we are more than just a physical body. The majority of who we are and what we can accomplish in life is unseen and being able to tap into those unseen aspects of the mental, emotional and spiritual world will have a greater possibility to assist in healing anything that ails the physical body. Learn to assess your client with four basic questions that will lead you to specific blockages based on what's going on in life. Then with an open heart learn what Naturopathic Reiki II has to offer that will grant you access to proficiency and longevity as a Naturopathic Reiki Therapist.

Chapter 2

Increasing Your
Personal Energy

Energy is motion, a constant vibration of varying degrees that moves the universe. Proficiency in Reiki and the work that guides the student in the second degree begins with a clear understanding of energy frequencies and how it effects the human body. This information is an attempt to assist the therapist to move from believing in the power of Reiki to "knowing" what Reiki does and how Reiki works. Reiki raises the human energy frequency. Humans have different levels of energy frequencies that are measured in bands of cycles per second (cps) or the equivalent is hertz (Hz). Using Reiki energy has been known to almost double the cps of the human body when used regularly.

The body's energy frequency is directly affected by what is present or lacking in the body in the way of nutrition, toxicity, and how a person lives. People who regulate their environment with positive and consistent quality in their physical, mental, emotional and spiritual bodies tend to vibrate at normal or higher frequencies.

A low-level frequency of less than 300 Hz shows up when the body is contaminated, diseased, stressed, obese, toxic or operating on irregular cycles according to the natural rhythms of human nature, for example when a person works overnight. Ideally when it is dark the human body is designed to be at rest to for its daily regenerative and cleansing processes. However, when the body is forced into this irregular cycle, its frequency is diminished.

Normal level frequency of 300 – 400 Hz is present in a person who is generally healthy by observing regular sleep patterns, a regular natural diet, and can deal with the normal stresses in life.

The Reiki level frequency of 400 – 800 Hz is an induced state that naturally increases the healing potential of the body. This frequency opens the many energy channels of the body through the chakras and meridians energizing the organ systems, the autonomic nervous system and the central nervous system which are all a part of the microcosm of universal presence.

The highest frequency vibrates above 800 Hz and is a state of spiritual mastery. At this level a person has mastered living a natural foods eating lifestyle, they have a daily ritual of meditation and they are living in alignment with nature according to the cycles of the earth. Stress and emotional habits become nonexistent and the person lives day to day with the tranquil peace of the highest self. This frequency is a rare experience.

This information is being introduced in the second degree of Naturopathic Reiki as preparation for taking your work in Reiki to the next level, especially in working with the symbols. There must be an understanding that the body is energy and energy is the body. There is no separation or isolation when Naturopathic Reiki becomes a health care service. The goal in energy mastery is to learn the flow of energy to increase the effects of Reiki through the second-degree tools.

Meridians

Imagine rivers of energy running down your arms to the tips of your fingers, down your legs to the tips of your toes, and from the top of your head down the front and back of your body. Imagine this constant flow of energy protection moving through you to supply every organ with the physical charge to fully function, the mental charge to do the correct job, the emotional charge to maintain balance and the spiritual charge to live long.

The energy channels in every living thing are called meridians. These lines of energy have been described and referenced for centuries in many different wellness therapies, especially those related to accessing unseen powers that people can utilize in healing. Although the meridians are labeled by a major organ, in naturopathy the focus is on the entire organ system that encompasses the noted organ. For example, the lung meridian would be relative to the whole respiratory system. Therefore, in Naturopathic Reiki when we work with the meridians it is a concentration of energy medicine to the entire organ system by way of the specific meridian of focus. The below diagrams are an overview of the lines of meridians.

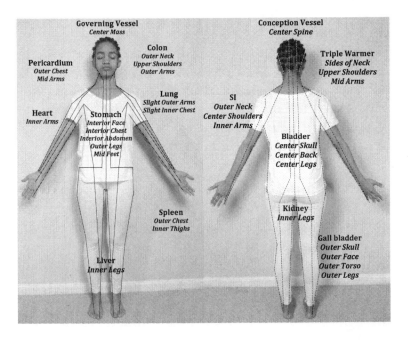

Each meridian has a starting and end point. Along each meridian are several energy vortexes called tsubos that also disseminate energy to and from the body similar to chakras, however, tsubos are the energy meters for the internal systems. In the second degree of Naturopathic Reiki, meridians are only introduced to understand the next level of energy functions and to make the student aware of the energy channels that are controlling what happens inside. It is in the third degree of Naturopathic Reiki where the health programs for working with the meridians are introduced as therapy.

The perfect way to maximize learning about energy once again is starting with yourself. The following exercises are time proven and innovative ways of increasing your personal energy flow. As you will see there is a balance between both breath exercises and physical exercises.

Energy Exercise 1: Meridian Stretches

To increase the personal internal energy that supplies your body's organ systems there are a series of meridian stretches to help. Each stretch covers two meridians. Working with these stretches should be a gradual process. You are encouraged to stay within your comfort zone. After you work with the stretches for some time and feel you can go further into the position do so but don't force yourself. The meridian stretches also originate from the Japanese energy medicine therapy, shiatsu. Note: Reiki and shiatsu are different systems, however, both have the foundation of using chi/ki as the source of healing.

Lungs and Large Intestine

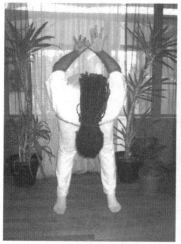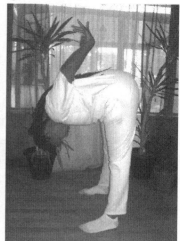

The two organs in the first stretch increases the oxygen supply to the body and stimulates the vital channel that removes solid waste. These are the two organs that end the nightly cleansing and regeneration process.

- ◆ Stand with your feet shoulder width apart keeping your feet parallel.
- ◆ Extend your hands behind your back and interlock your thumbs.
- ◆ On your next exhale slowly lean forward in a bend toward your feet.
- ◆ Extend your interlocked hands up behind your back and hold the stretch at a comfortable point.
- ◆ Breathe deeply, no bouncing; just a deep stretch.
- ◆ You will feel a gentle stretch all along the back of your legs from the ankles up.
- ◆ Release the stretch on an inhale, relaxing your knees while coming up.
- ◆ Release your interlocked thumbs and relax your stance.
- ◆ Repeat two more times.

Stomach and Spleen

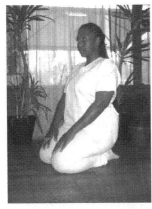 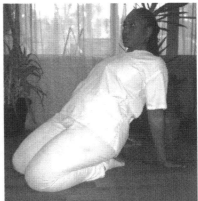

These two organs have their optimal functioning time during the day. The spleen is the body's storage tank for the daily blood supply that's needed for increased physical activity. The stomach is the mechanism that breaks down the food particles to supply the cells with energy for the entire body. These two organs get you moving.

- ◆ Begin this floor stretch sitting comfortably with legs folded beneath you, back straight and hands resting on your thighs.
- ◆ On an inhale begin to lower the top part of your body as far back as you can comfortably go. (*This modified version pictured here is for beginners.*)
- ◆ Support your upper body with your hands to the floor if needed. More advanced students can rest their entire back on the floor and stretch your arms straight up above your head.
- ◆ On an exhale slowly bring the body back forward to the upright position. Back straight with hands resting on thighs.
- ◆ Repeat two more times.

Heart and Small Intestine

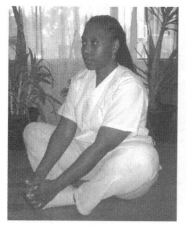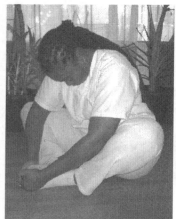

Two more organs that are vital to supplying the blood and nutrients to the body are the next meridian stretch. The optimal functioning time for the heart and small intestine are mid-morning to mid-day. Use this stretch to tone the energy of the heart and revitalize the proficiency of nutrient assimilation.

- ◆ Sit on your seat bottom, back straight, with soles of feet together.
- ◆ Take a few deep breaths and relax your gaze.
- ◆ With hands clasped around the toes, on the exhale lean forward at the waist as far as you can go to remain comfortable.
- ◆ Be mindful to keep your bottom on the floor.
- ◆ Feel the gentle stretch through your back, inner thighs and arms.
- ◆ Release the stretch on an inhale as you bring the body back up to the straight back position.
- ◆ Release the toes and relax.
- ◆ Repeat two more times.

Bladder and Kidneys

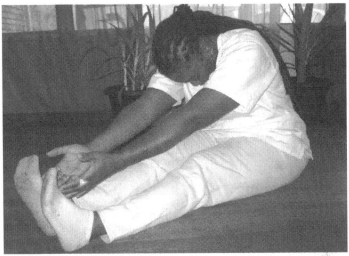

Now we are moving towards the end of the work day and the body is preparing for rest and regeneration. First it cleanses out the liquid waste through the kidneys and bladder. Although this stretch is very common in the world of yoga and exercise, it is also a valuable addition to the world of meridians.

- Sit on the floor with a straight back and legs extended in front of you.
- If you can't sit with straight legs, it is ok to bend your knees to a comfortable level.
- Take a few deep breaths and on an exhale, bend the body forward towards the feet extending the hands beyond the soles.
- Breathe into this position, without bouncing, and feel the gentle stretch from your ankle to your neck.
- Release the stretch on an inhale as you bring your body back up to a straight back, resting your hands on your thighs.
- Repeat two more times.

Pericardium and Triple Heater

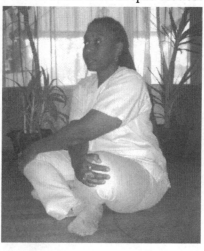

These two meridians are governed by a series of organs and strong energy centers in the body, they begin your night process internally. The pericardium is the sex center which heightens the function of the reproductive system. This is why the best time for sex is between 7 pm and 9 pm. (See *Holistic Sexuality: The Practical Guide to Sexual Healing by K. Akua Gray* for additional information.) The triple heater supplies the body with its heat source while the body rests and "burns off" the waste products of the day. There is one organ in the triple heater, the liver, which also has its individual functioning time in the next segment, and the two energy centers that generate heat in the body are the solar plexus and the hara. The solar plexus is a chakra, (refer to *Naturopathic Reiki I: Opening the Way also by K. Akua Gray* for a full explanation on the solar plexus) and the hara is an energy vortex that rests at the center of the body, located three fingers width below the naval. The hara is considered the energy point where all movement of the body originates.

- Sit either in the half lotus or full lotus crossed legged position with back straight.
- Take a few deep breaths.
- Crisscross arms and grasp the opposite knees.
- On an exhale lean forward as far as you can comfortably go.
- Feel the arms, fingers, back and legs.
- Breathe in and spread the shoulder blades to accentuate the entire triple heater system.
- Breathe out and relax.
- On the next inhale sit up straight.
- Release the arms and take a few deep breaths.
- Repeat two more times.

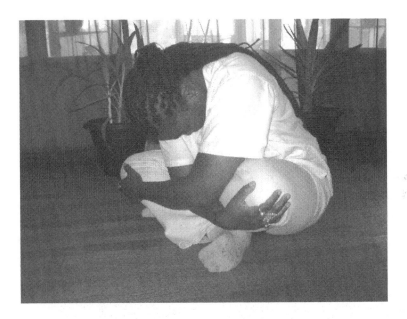

Gallbladder and Liver

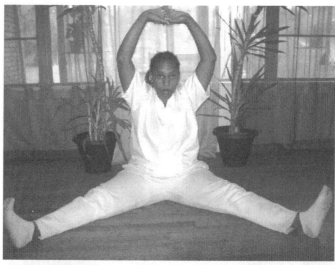

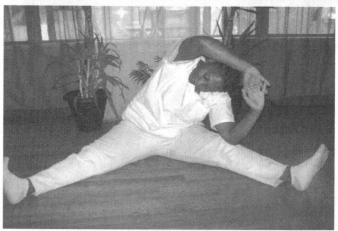

The gallbladder and liver work together while you are sleeping every night to clean the blood, manufacture solid waste, and restore life and energy to the cells. The process of cleansing and regeneration alone is why getting the proper amount of sleep every night is necessary. The liver and sleep help keep you younger longer.

- Sitting on the floor with a straight back open your legs wide but comfortable.
- Take a few deep breaths.
- On an inhale extend your hands over your head and interlock your fingers.
- With fingers still interlocked flip the palms upward towards the ceiling.
- On the next exhale lean the body down the left leg as far as you can comfortably go.
- Feel the stretch along your right side and through the legs.
- On an inhale come back to center.
- Take a deep breath and on the exhale, lean down the right leg as far as you can go comfortably.
- Feel the stretch along your left side and through the legs.
- On an inhale come back to center.
- Repeat two more times.
- After the third time come back to center on an inhale and turn your interlocked hands over.
- Release the arms down on the last exhale.

This energy exercise routine will take about fifteen minutes of your day. It is a way to start your day, especially if you have Reiki clients to service. When you perform these stretches regularly, you are preparing the internal energy of your own body to fully function at its maximum capacity. Taking care of yourself is vital to helping to take care of others. An added benefit to the meridian stretches is their ability to align you with the internal elements air, fire, water, earth and spirit. We explore the elements at its deepest level in third degree Naturopathic Reiki.

Energy Exercise 2: Fire Breaths

Fire Breaths are one of the easiest ways to reach a level of high energy. Fire Breaths are a method of trance induction that comes directly from the hara. These quick pumps of breath in and out the lungs through the nostrils is done in a lotus sitting position with the legs crossed or sitting straight up in a chair with feet flat on the floor.

The transcendental state that is achieved with mastering this breath work is mediumistic trance. When one reaches this level of trance, it opens the portals to the subconscious mind. This level of consciousness is where the will of manifestation is activated to affect the physical realm of existence. While in mediumistic trance it is a good time to see your life as you want it to be. It is a time to send focus to achieving your goals. It is a good time to send healing energy to your body to eliminate dis-ease and imbalances.

Using Fire Breaths to enter mediumistic trance also forms a protective force field around you by activating the entire chakra system.

Fire Breaths physically tightens your abdomen, mentally brings you quickly to a trance state for meditation, quiets the emotions and spiritually allows you access to the astral realm to make an impact on your learning processes and ability to manifest your will during meditation. Ideally you can comfortably do one hundred Fire Breaths per minute. The most affective number of Fire Breaths in one meditation period is one thousand. However, the novice must gradually work up to this level over a period of months.

about 100 breaths per minute

Energy Exercise 3: Chop It Up

A wonderful yet simple energy opening exercise in self-manipulation is a common Qi gong exercise that allows you to stimulate the energy in every part of the body inside and out. Basically, you give your body taps and chops starting from the top of the body down through the legs to "awaken" the meridians.

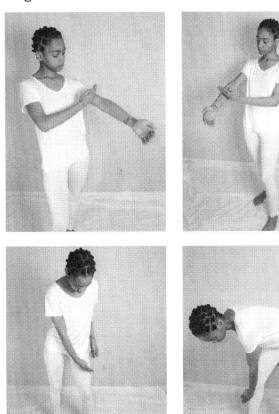

Energy Exercise 4: Breath of Innocence

Growing in Naturopathic Reiki means developing new skills to nurture your body, mind and spirit. We will explore meditation as one of these skills to prepare you to be a proficient second degree therapist in later chapters. Again, we return to the breath as one of the ways to gain instant relaxation with vitality from life's primary resource, air. The Breath of Innocence is not only a benefit, but a requirement for those seeking full energy rejuvenation. The source of proper breathing takes us back to the day we were born. Babies breathe in the purest of forms by filling their abdomens, then their chest and finally their nasal cavities all in one inhale. The exhale is also naturally in the reverse order. This Breath of Innocence as I like to refer to it, immediately returns the mind, body, soul and emotions to a state of peace. Let's try it.

Sitting in a comfortable position either on the floor or in a chair, hands resting on your lap, and eyes closed, begin Mindful Breathing. (See *Naturopathic Reiki I: Opening the Way by K. Akua Gray for* the instructions of this breath technique.)

Once your Mindful Breathing has become rhythmic, on the next inhale expand the abdomen to full capacity, then continue to breathe in to fill the chest with air and without holding the breath, exhale slowly first from the chest and then the abdomen and repeat 5 – 10 more times until you feel comfortable.

Finally, inhale filling the abdomen, the chest and then the nasal cavity and without a break between breaths, slowly exhale in reverse order. Repeat 5 – 10 times until you feel comfortable and completely relaxed.

The Breath of Innocence should be performed regularly. It can be used to increase your energy for Reiki, studying, prayer, yoga, detox, channeling, relaxation and when you need an air of peace.

Energy Exercise 5: Sun Gazing

The sun and its life-giving energy has many references throughout the second degree of Naturopathic Reiki. To consciously connect with this powerful star in our solar system is the foundation to internalizing the use of the Reiki symbols and the healthcare programs that we will learn about in later chapters.

Sun gazing in its most innocent form is something that most of us did as children. Of course not knowing the benefits of sun exposure, we just wanted to be outside to feel the air and adventure that nature had to give us. However, sun gazing to access higher energy levels in the body is slightly different than play time in the sun. Note: If you are not used to being in the sun make sure to gradually work your way up to full exposure and always hydrate before and after this exercise.

- Find a quiet space outside where you won't be disturbed for at least fifteen minutes.
- In a full sun area either sit on the earth or in a comfortable chair with your feet flat to the ground.
- Begin with Gassho Breath for a few moments to regulate the breath and relax.
- When you are ready turn your face up to the sun with eyes closed and feel the rays on your skin for a few seconds. Repeat two more times.
- Next lie down or stand up and stretch out your arms to the side in an act of opening the body to the sun for a few seconds.

- Finally place your Reiki hands over your eyes and with small cracks between your fingers gaze directly at the sun and let the power fill your retina. Note: Do not look at the sun without the protective shield of your Reiki hands.
- Repeat two more times.

Each time that you practice sun gazing, you will find that you can stay in the sun longer. This exercise is proven to energize the central nervous system, the melanin neurological system, strengthen the bones and fortify positive thinking.

Chapter 2 Summary

Increasing your personal energy is vital when you begin to provide Naturopathic Reiki as a professional service. As a therapist, the energy frequency that you channel will be a unique experience for every client. To prepare for the physical, mental, emotional and spiritual work it is required that you fortify yourself by raising your energy frequency with personal breath therapy and physical therapy. Each exercise is designed to be an extensive presentation of self-love that can be used as long as Reiki lives in you.

Chapter 3

The Reiki Symbols

There are three standard symbols in the second degree of Reiki and two additional ancient symbols that also provide positive effects on a naturopathic level. The use of symbols date back to antiquity and as one of the first forms of written communication. For this reason, symbols can produce energy frequencies that words cannot express. A simple symbol can generate thought patterns that bring about actions, sound waves, and cellular vibrations that can captivate the mental, physical, emotional and spiritual consciousness of a person instantaneously.

Think about the symbols that you encounter every day. In modern society, we call them logos. Even without words these logos/symbols may have a direct effect on your actions, mood or what you desire in the spur of the moment. This knowledge of what symbols can do was mastered by the ancient Egyptians of Kemet, who built an entire civilization around the mastery of symbols. And because they were the teachers of all civilizations after them the remnants of this knowledge has had a trickle down affect all the way to the twentieth century.

Twentieth century symbolism in Reiki is a beautiful representation of the ancient past coming to life for the spiritual, mental, emotional and physical care of humanity. The Reiki symbols were formed to contain power, spark creativity, move energy matter, and guard mystical information. To awaken an ability as it relates to energy medicine is to bring life to a pure frequency that is already present but dormant. Once an ability is fully awakened it then channels and aligns itself to a similar vibration to draw lower vibrations up to a higher frequency. Finally, when all vibrational levels have merged into oneness, only then can the mystical information to maintain that frequency be disseminated on a cellular level and become part of the molecular memory. Reiki symbols are spiritual tools to help you connect, focus, and use Reiki to its fullest capacity.

Drawing the Symbols

Reiki symbols are traditionally drawn mentally. The mind is faster than the hand, because the motion of the hand must come through the mind. Therefore, to visualize a symbol facilitates instant results. However, because people are creatures of ritual, the ritualistic drawing of the symbols is also taught to the novice to help impress upon the memory the detail of accuracy as a formal way of learning the Reiki symbols. The Reiki symbols can be used for every treatment that you provide or only during specific treatments. Always draw the Reiki symbols from left to right.

- Draw a Reiki symbol with your finger on the palm of your hands to activate Reiki.
- Draw the Reiki symbol with your whole hand (in the air) to exaggerate the size of the symbol to cover a large area.
- Draw them directly over the recipient's body before a treatment.
- Draw the symbols over a particular area of the body to concentrate the energy that the Reiki symbol represents.
- Draw them at the end of a treatment to close out the therapy.

The Reiki symbols are also empowered by words called mantras. Mantras hold mystical vibrations that effect the frequencies of energy. For example, two of the most used mantra in the world today originated in ancient Kemet and ancient Dravidian India. "Amen" is a word of power that solidifies the essence of all things seen and unseen that manifest in the world. It has been adopted by every major religion for over the past 6,000 years. Also, the mantra "OM" has gained popularity for the last 5,000 years as a mantra that represents the sound of source energy, the universe. Like these mainstream mantras, the mantras of the Reiki symbols will represent for the Naturopathic Reiki therapist words of power to be chanted, recited, and spoken within the heart and mind to add fuel to the movement of healing energy.

CHO KU REI
choe koo ray
The Power Symbol

The first Reiki symbol is a visual representation of the essence of the universe. Acknowledgement of the divine cycle of power that we live in is the beginning of understanding Cho ku rei. All manifestations and awareness are known to come from one source of energy. The foundation emblem in Cho ku rei is similar to the governing vessel that controls the microcosm of the human body, the spine. Also, the second component of the symbol is a spiral. Everything in the physical world is represented by a cycle. Cycles are spirals of times and presence that keep the flow of energy constant. Thus, the spiral that is represented in the Cho ku rei symbol calls forth the core of universal power each time it is used.

The mantra Cho ku rei as source energy originates in pure movement. It is the activator of the will of the divine therefore, it is associated with the solar plexus. If you recall, the solar plexus empowers the soul to exert and use power for purpose and progress. To visualize Cho ku rei with consistency will empower you as a therapist to move instantaneously towards those things that are in alignment with the divine cycle of life.

When you see Cho ku rei think,
"the will of divine energy."

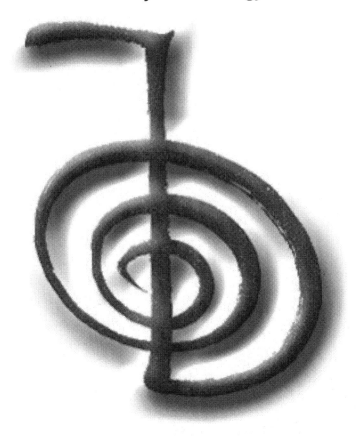

To draw Cho ku rei start on the left and draw the rod of life giving energy from top to bottom, then going counter clockwise spiral to the center of the rod.

Reiki Power Moves

A Reiki power move using Cho ku rei is a list of various ways to enhance the Naturopathic Reiki experience for your client. These power moves also provide the experience you need as a therapist to learn all that can be done with the second degree Reiki symbols. In Naturopathic Reiki, each power move is categorized by the health aspect that the move is best used for per the needs of your client.

Physical
Cho ku rei is the most versatile of the second degree Reiki symbols. It can be used in every type of therapy and health program.

Cho ku rei helps to improve the physical and material state if there are tangible things that need to change in your life or with your client.

Cho ku rei can help reduce pain. Cho ku rei taps directly into source energy and works to elevate the low frequency of pain.

Draw Cho ku rei over all personal care items to increase the energy frequency of anything that will be put on or in the body.

Draw Cho ku rei over food before cooking and eating. Most food and water go through a series of processes to reach the shopping centers and the dining table. Anytime something is processed, it loses components of its original nutritional value. Although Cho ku rei does not replace nutrients, it can raise the energy frequency of processed food and water so that the body's energy level is not depleted from processed consumption.

Mental
When your energy is low give yourself a treatment, draw Cho ku rei down your body, and run Reiki for five -minutes.

Cho ku rei is an excellent sleep aid. To relax the mind completely, visualize, chant or run Reiki with the power symbol right before bed.

Cho ku rei enhances the unifying nature of the mind to recover from judgement, peer stress, self-degrading thoughts, and doubt.

Use Cho ku rei with clients who have a hard time dealing with the pressures of life.

Use Cho ku rei with clients that are indecisive about choices that need to be made for their progress and purpose.

Emotional
Cho ku rei is energy protection. Use it to dissipate fear and fortify courage.

Cho ku rei is an excellent symbol and mantra to use to calm anger, sadness and despondency. These emotions are barriers to a person's peace of mind. When negative emotional behavior dominates a person's life they find it difficult to rest, nurture and be nurtured.

Cho ku rei helps to create a better mood and lifts the spirit. There is a certain serenity and joy that comes with empowerment. To be empowered with the knowledge that things will get better despite whatever may be happening in life helps a person to keep moving forward.

Draw Cho ku rei in therapies where your client needs clarity in their actions.

Draw Cho ku rei to level out an emotional situation. Cho ku rei can be a safety net to absorb emotional outburst during therapy.

Spiritual
Cho ku rei helps align human energy with the natural rhythm of the earth. To be in alignment with the cycles of existence preserves the body, increases the brain function, balances the emotions and sets the spirit at peace.

You can use Cho ku rei at the start of all healing sessions to bring the highest source of good energy for the therapy.

Draw Cho ku rei into the corners of any room that needs spiritual cleaning. To cleanse a room, draw or visualize Cho ku rei in the corners or on the walls, floor, and ceiling while intending that the room be cleaned and filled with energies of love and compassion.

Cho ku rei can be used to charge spiritual tools such as crystals, wands, and grids.

You can draw it over your client at the end of a session to seal and stabilize the healing.

Cho ku rei is the symbol to use when Reiki is to be run for an extended period of time, such as hours, days, weeks or months. Reiki has no limit on the amount of time that you can channel and send the energy, for example, if a person is involved with a long term medical regimen such as cancer treatment. It would be good to keep Reiki flowing to and through that person until re-mission is confirmed.

Cho Ku Rei Affirmations*

The mantra Cho ku rei should be internalized, applied and mastered by the therapist as a power tool not only for your life but for the success and effectiveness of all the Reiki work you will do for others. The following af-firmations were created to live with and share to make the existence of Cho ku rei a way of life.

When you say Cho ku rei feel, "the will of divine energy."

- ♦ I am a servant to the divine truth and a spiritual warrior against all illusion. Cho ku rei.
- ♦ I free my soul from ignorance. I am not my body. I am the infinite peace of the universe. Cho ku rei.
- ♦ I recognize that I am divine. As divine energy I am the cause that all things exist. I will live today like the energy that sustains all things. Cho ku rei.
- ♦ When my spirit leads me in my first mind thoughts, I will follow. Cho ku rei.
- ♦ When my spirit leads me to speak words of light, I will let them be heard. Cho ku rei.
- ♦ When my spirit leads me to change for my greater good, I will walk according to my purpose. Cho ku rei.
- ♦ When my spirit leads me to nourish my body with the goodness of the Earth, I will choose life and enjoy. I will live like I KNOW who I am. Cho ku rei.

- I have a unique vibrational alignment with the universe. We have all manifested in the physical to be an experience to the world. My life is a pattern of successes that brings me an unshakable peace. Cho ku rei.
- I appreciate the virtues of my soul: knowledge, service and respect. Cho ku rei.
- I am conscious of divine energy in everything I do, in every word I say and in everyone I meet. Cho ku rei.
- I will do it. Cho ku rei.

Cho Ku Rei Chants

To chant is to impress upon the spirit a permanent change that instructs the mind to respond and live a particular way. Chanting is also an ancient system of remembering, guiding and empowering groups and individuals to harmonize with the spirit of nature to activate the fullness of life. In Naturopathic Reiki to chant the mantras will align you as the therapist and your clients to the highest good of any situation or imbalance. Use these chants in private meditation time, during therapy, or as a personal exercise for your client to take with them and use for their own spiritual development.

- Cho ku rei is my power to live.
- Cho ku rei moves me in the world.
- Cho ku rei is my personal power.
- Cho ku rei heals me.
- Cho ku rei is my infinite source.

The Cho Ku Rei Empowerment Plan

As in the first degree of Naturopathic Reiki you were encouraged to work on empowering yourself with the new information to ensure your seriousness about taking on the responsibility that comes with using energy medicine with the Naturopathic Reiki Level I - 21 Day Clearing. In the second degree of Naturopathic Reiki there is a 7 Day Empowerment Plan for each symbol to help you get acquainted with the most important tools.

Day 1 – For morning or evening meditation, center yourself with the Gassho breath. When you are relaxed and ready chant the mantra Cho ku rei seven times while visualizing the symbol going into each of your chakras. Give yourself a short Reiki treatment to close out the meditation.

Day 2 – Repeat day 1. In your Naturopathic Reiki journal practice writing the symbol Cho ku rei ten times and answer the following questions.
- How do I define power?
- What areas or situations do I need to bring more spiritual power into my life?
- How much of this power am I willing to share with others?

Day 3 – Repeat day 1. Practice charging by physically drawing Cho ku rei around the room that you are in or the space around you if you are outside and with each drawing say, "It is the will of divine energy."

Day 4 – Repeat day 1. Mentally draw Cho ku rei and will it to cover your entire body. Then mentally draw Cho ku rei again and visualize it covering the body of another person who you know needs power to change something in their life. Conclude the visualization with, "It is the will of divine energy."

Day 5 - For morning or evening meditation center yourself with the Gassho breath. When you are relaxed and ready chant the mantra Cho ku rei thirty times while visualizing the symbol going into the throat chakra ten times, the brow chakra ten times and the crown chakra ten times. Think about one of the areas or situations you wrote about in your journal for Cho ku rei day 2 and visualize Cho ku rei and the solution. Give yourself at least a fifteen-minute Reiki treatment to close out the meditation.

Day 6 – Repeat day 5 using a different area or situation. This Cho ku rei meditation can be used for as many days as it takes to manifest the change.

Day 7 – For morning or evening meditation center yourself with the Gassho breath. When you are relaxed and ready chant the mantra Cho ku rei thirty times while visualizing the symbol going into throat chakra ten times, the brow chakra ten times and the crown chakra ten times. Give Cho ku rei to the world. Send it out to touch the hearts, minds, bodies and lives of all existence. Then visualize Cho ku rei at your heart chakra and bless it with a short Reiki treatment. Now send it down to each of the lower chakras, the solar plexus, the sacral and the root with a short Reiki treatment. When you feel relaxed and complete send Cho ku rei down through the soles of your feet and into the earth to bless the world from within. You and Cho ku rei are now complete.

SEI HE KI
say hay key
The Harmony, Emotional, and Mental Healing Symbol

The second Reiki symbol taps into the invisible human nature through the limbic system and the central nervous system. Sei he ki is about feeling the balance of life. Feeling is what creates the awareness of the physical connection to the world. Feeling also creates the mental and emotional awareness to imbalances which provokes all healing. The symbol of Sei he ki has a likeness to human form as a reminder that although we see the physical, the majority of the balance in life comes from those aspects of the unseen in humanity such as harmony, the emotions and the mind.

The mantra Sei he ki aligns the physical body with the invisible life of man's experience through the emotions, which has a tranquilizing effect. Sei he ki calms negative anxious energy and negative emotions that are congesting the mind and body.

Sei he ki's source is in the heart chakra. It is the energy center that vibrates unconditional expression of one of the most powerful energies that people use in every relationship, love. Often that love is expressed as fear when there is emotional immaturity that does not recognize the abundance of the universe. Love and hate also share a familiar space in emotional dysfunction, because most people are unaware that the two feelings are polarities of balance stemming from the same energy. However, spiritual ascension of the individual alters the thought processes to the former because love vibrates at a higher frequency. Sei he ki is this type of awareness personified and applied through Naturopathic Reiki.

Emotions are a major focus for Naturopathic Reiki healing because of their addictive nature spawned by the biochemical reactions in the central nervous system when they occur.

When you see Sei he ki think, "live in peace."

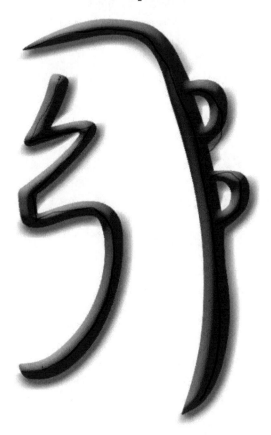

To draw Sei he ki, start on the left and draw the "face" first from top to bottom, then come back up to the top and draw the "head" down to the "neck", and finally the two humps on the back.

To visualize Sei he ki with consistency will empower you as a Naturopathic Reiki therapist to move in and out of your emotional episodes instantaneously without overloading the mind, body and nervous system with excessive biochemical feedback. In other words, you will learn to feel your emotions for the allotted three seconds that it takes to process and then release it and focus on the lesson that is coming from why the emotion happened in the first place. Emotions are biochemical teaching tools to help us learn from our environment. It is the mind that carries emotions on for long periods of time disturbing your peace.

Reiki Power Moves
for Mental and Emotional Healing

A Reiki power move using Sei he ki is used when the lower chakras which are primarily affected by the emotions show evidence of stress and imbalance. When you consult with your client at the beginning of the appointment some of these issues may come out, and if nothing is mentioned specifically by the client, you will be able to do a chakra reading to determine any blockages.

Mental
When you are emotionally unstable for more than three seconds give yourself a treatment, draw Sei he ki down your body, and give yourself a five-minute tranquilizer.

Sei he ki is used to lessen the symptoms of depression. However, since depression is a medical diagnosis this terminology must come from your client. Beware not to diagnose any disease.

Sei he ki can be used in the chakras with the intention to balance excessive emotions. People tend to hold on to emotions like anger, sadness and fear which paralyze their ability to move forward in life.

Sei he ki is also used to maintain mental balance when working on keeping a positive attitude in the face of challenges and obstacles.

Sei he ki can dissipate bad vibes and negativity. Sometimes it's the negative environment that infects the mind of your clients. Chanting Sei he ki is an excellent resource to create positive outcomes from encountering negativity.

Sei he ki can improve and assist with memory. Place your hand on your head and draw Sei he ki. As you run Reiki say to yourself: *"I will remember ..."* then just relax. Reiki helps align the conscious mind to the memory. This works because Reiki helps you relax so that information can resurface. Reiki can help your conscious mind to access to information from all the data in your brain.

Sei he ki also helps with releasing bad habits. It is the mind that allows the biochemical dependency of doing things that a person knows is not good for them. For example, smoking, drinking alcohol and taking recreational drugs. Once the mind accepts the physical reaction of the substance, the chemistry of the body solidifies the deal with addiction. Sei he ki is an excellent addition to any type of detox program.

When relationships are stressed, dysfunctional or unhealthy, Sei he ki can improve the understanding of the individuals who are seeking harmony.

Trauma can destroy the mind. Sei he ki is used in all cases of trauma. It moves the energy of the memory to a neutral zone in the neurological functions of the brain and allows for peace to replace the pain.

Unhealthy attachments also cause mental imbalances. People force themselves to survive constant mental and emotional assaults in their relationships with family, friends, co-workers, employers and sometimes strangers. Sei he ki can help reverse the effects of such unwanted behavior by making it easier for the client to release the relationships in a peaceful manner. Sei he ki invokes courage.

Emotional
Sei he ki aligns the body with the higher frequency emotions such as serenity, joy, happiness, however, these emotions also are only experienced for three seconds in a healthy individual.

Sei he ki is used to invoke compassion to help others. Compassion is an emotion of action. Sei he ki moves you to action.

Sei he ki enhances your ability to love yourself. It is said in holistic health the you can only give what you have. The best way to facilitate healing in any capacity is to first provide that healing for yourself. Taking care of yourself in the best way, with the best things and at all times prepares you to share that same zest and sweetness of life with others.

Sei he ki opens the way to loving others that is aligned with their higher good. This means teaching the mind and spirit to accept itself. Use Sei he ki to help clients connect fully with the souls of others.

Sei he ki will assist with unblocking feelings for a free flow of energy to experience true emotions. Sei he ki opens the energy channels of the limbic system for healthy emotional expression.

If there is a situation of argument or disagreement, imagine Sei he ki between the two people. Sei he ki will filter the energy exchange and assist in creating harmony, peace, and understanding.

Sei he ki is used to reduce emotional stress. Until a person takes the time needed to mature their emotional state of mind. Sei he ki can quickly and temporarily calm emotional stress.

Sei he ki restores high energy when a person has been emotionally drained by an event. What we see and hear affects the mind and body and cause temporary moments of depression that brings the whole energy level down.

Sei he ki is used to assist in self-programming for emotional healing. When a person is ready to enter into an emotional healing program the Sei he ki mantra and symbol are a dynamic meditation focus that will solidify healing and longevity.

When protection is needed draw Sei he ki around yourself and others and affirm: *"Sei he ki protects me with divine love and wisdom." "Sei he ki protects you with divine love and wisdom."*

Sei he ki Affirmations

Affirmations are a powerful tool to achieve goals. Simply repeat a positive phrase in your mind, or write it on paper. Repetition is the key and the mantra Sei he ki is used to empower your affirmations. The combination deeply embeds the affirmation in the subconscious mind.

When you say Sei he ki feel the peace come over you.

- ♦ I forgive my enemy thoughts. I will only uplift myself from this day forward. Sei he ki.
- ♦ Money in life is relative. Relate to it as needed. Sei he ki.
- ♦ I am not afraid to speak my truth today; it frees my mind from attachments. Sei he ki.
- ♦ I consciously choose to be at peace today. This state of enchantment is the essence of my true being. Sei he ki.
- ♦ I am my own guide to perfect peace. Sei he ki.
- ♦ I only have room for light and life fulfilling purpose in my world. Sei he ki.
- ♦ I care for my mind with positive, powerful, and pure thoughts. Sei he ki.
- ♦ I will control my mouth by controlling my mind. Sei he ki.
- ♦ Love is the divine energy connection of all things seen and unseen and it is the force that fuels my life of freedom. Sei he ki.
- ♦ I consciously think about the ripple effect of what I say and do. Sei he ki.

The mantra Sei he ki should be internalized, applied and mastered by the therapist as a power tool not only for your life but for the success and effectiveness of all the Naturopathic Reiki work you will do for others.

Sei he ki Hand Positions to Eliminate Emotional Organ Stress

The organs can be directly affected by excessive emotions. The biochemical releases of emotions from the brain change the energy levels of the organs and reduce the organ's ability to fight disease as well as cause physical damage to the organ. The following hand positions are executed in alignment with the nerve endings of the face that are relative to the specific organ. Since the face areas are small, the use of a finger or two is all that is needed to administer Naturopathic Reiki.

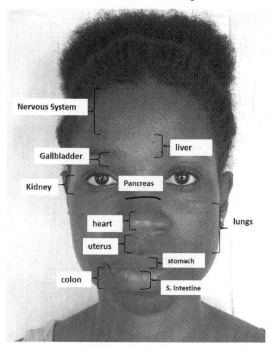

Intestines

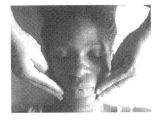

Stress

Stomach

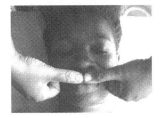

Anxiety

Kidneys

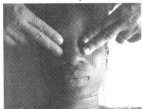

Fear
Anxiety
Confusion

Liver

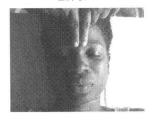

Anger
Frustration
Jealousy

Spleen

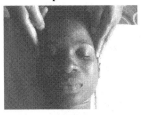

Panic
Shock

Heart

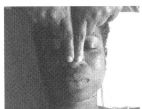

Sadness
Depression

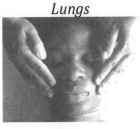

Lungs

Worry
Grief
Sorrow

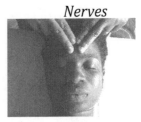

Nerves

Guilt
Denial

Naturopathic Reiki can also be administered directly to the internal organs based on their actual location in the body to also relieve emotional stress.

Intestines

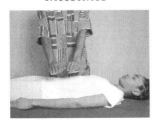

Stress

Stomach

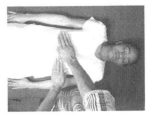

Anxiety

Kidneys

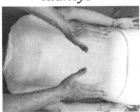

Fear
Anxiety
Confusion

Liver

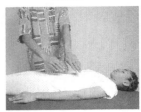

Anger
Frustration
Jealousy

Spleen

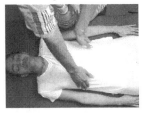

Panic
Shock

Heart

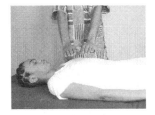

Sadness
Depression

Lungs

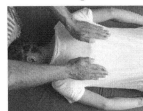

Worry
Grief
Sorrow

Nerves

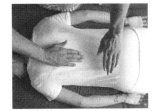

Guilt

Emotional stress has the potential to destroy life. Unfortunately the ways to bring balance to life's emotional responses are only taught in schools of wellness. The larger society and it's institutions of education, media and medicine only offer confirmation of emotional dysfunction as the normal way for people to respond and relate to each other. However, we are seeing in the twenty-first century an increase in the number of schools and institutes that promote, teach and provide excellent examples of how emotions were designed to benefit human nature for its highest good.

Sei he ki Chants

The Sei he ki chant is to invoke the invisible power of healing for the mind. In Naturopathic Reiki to chant the mantras will align you as the therapist and your clients to the highest good of any situation or imbalance. Use these chants in private meditation time, during therapy, or as a personal exercise for your client to take with them and use for their own emotional and mental development.

 ♦ Sei he ki heals my heart.
 ♦ My thoughts are pure. Sei he ki .
 ♦ I let go freely. Sei he ki.
 ♦ There is joy in Sei he ki.
 ♦ Sei he ki lightens all darkness.

The Sei he ki Empowerment Plan

In addition to the 7 Day work in Cho ku rei, there is also a 7 Day Empowerment Plan for Sei he ki to help you get acquainted with using this symbol for the great works that you will do.

Day 1 – For morning or evening meditation center yourself with the Gassho breath. When you are relaxed and ready chant the mantra Sei he ki four times while visualizing the symbol going into each of your upper chakras, the heart, throat, brow and crown. Give yourself a short Reiki treatment to close out the meditation.

Day 2 – Repeat day 1. In your Naturopathic Reiki journal practice writing the Sei he ki symbol ten times. Also recall in your journal any negative emotional episodes you experienced or witnessed recently that left you feeling uneasy. After you have written the summary visualize a different outcome and give yourself a ten-minute self-treatment.

Make a commitment to yourself as you go through your day to actively think about your emotional responses to any situations that may arouse your emotions negatively for more than three seconds. For example, do you have to respond when your anger is aroused or can you develop the peaceful intent to learn from every interaction? Use Sei he ki to help you by visualizing it or chanting the mantra.

Day 3 – Repeat day 1. Journal how you did yesterday in responding to any negative emotions. Were you successful in living in the peacefulness of Sei he ki?

Day 4 – Repeat day 1. Mentally draw Sei he ki and cover your heart with it. Then mentally draw Sei he ki again and visualize it attaching to the heart of another person who you know needs the power to heal from emotional turmoil in their life. Conclude the visualization with the words, "Live in peace."

Day 5 - For morning or evening meditation center yourself with the Gassho breath. When you are relaxed and ready chant the mantra Sei he ki forty times while visualizing the symbol going into the heart chakra ten times, the throat chakra ten times, the brow chakra ten times and the crown chakra ten times. Visualize the perfect situation for you in life right now, in terms of your relationships, employment/business, and what will help you to grow to your highest potential. Give yourself at least a fifteen-minute Reiki treatment to close out the meditation.

Day 6 – Repeat day 5. This Sei he ki meditation can be used for as many days as it takes to manifest the change.

Day 7 – For morning or evening meditation center yourself with the Gassho breath. When you are relaxed and ready chant the mantra Sei he ki forty times while visualizing the symbol going into the heart chakra ten times, throat chakra ten times, the brow chakra ten times and the crown chakra ten times. Then visualize Sei he ki streaming from your heart chakra and healing the world from emotional imbalance. When you feel relaxed and complete send Sei he ki all around your body in a beautiful golden light that covers you from head to toe. You and Sei he ki are now complete.

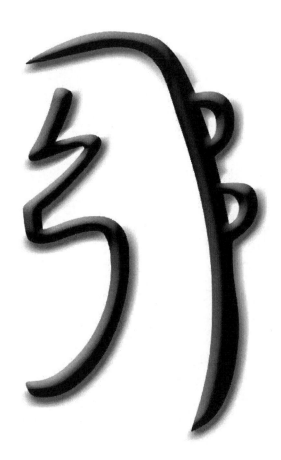

HON SHA ZE SHO NEN
(hone shah zay show nane)
The Distance Healing Symbol

The third Reiki symbol is mastered through an understanding of metaphysics. When it is internalized by the Naturopathic Reiki therapist that the universe is an unending multidimensional connection of energy then Hon sha ze sho nen becomes real, accessible and a reliable tool in Naturopathic Reiki therapy. To physically touch the soul is a powerful endeavor, however for the Naturopathic Reiki therapist that effectively uses Hon sha ze sho nen it is a regular occurrence of channeling intended for the recipient's highest good. A viable example of this energy is the beautiful and mighty sun. The ball of fire is 92.96 million miles from the earth however, when you walk outside in its rays you feel the energy and power of this magnificent star right on your skin. This is the same way that Hon sha ze sho nen has no limits on distance, time or space.

Hon sha ze sho nen has its source in the brow chakra. Like intuition it connects easily with those things that are unseen. Distance healing can be executed for short or extremely long distances. Hon sha ze sho nen is used to connect to past life situations that need healing, current life changes and to ease anxieties about the future. As people, we are always thinking about one of the three moments of time related to living. Although we are taught in the study of metaphysics to focus with an open heart on the present; we can't help but plan for tomorrow and remember the past. Since this is our normal way of existing, there is only a problem when thoughts of the past and future disturb our peace of mind. Hon sha ze sho nen is the spiritual essence of divine energy that restores that balance.

The nature of human existence is a state of peace. Whether the individual has internalized it or not, inevitably everyone wants to be peaceful. Peace is a state of balance and equilibrium that allows us to manage everything in life.

When you see Hon sha ze sho nen think, "eternal omni presence."

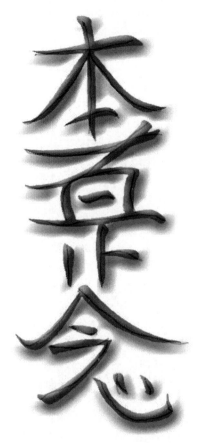

To draw Hon sha ze sho nen start at the top of the symbol and again go from left to right with each stroke. This will be demonstrated by your teacher.

This symbol is the most complicated of the Reiki symbols but can be easy to learn with practice. Start with one stroke, repeat that stroke until you learn it and continue adding another stroke until you are able to write the complete symbol. Also remember that you can activate the Reiki function by direct intention without drawing or visualizing the symbol, however, it is crucial for you to learn it.

The mantra Hon sha ze sho nen is used to stop the world and all its chatter. When Hon sha ze sho nen is spoken it immediately breaks down the illusion of space, time and distance and opens a portal for pure energy to flow, restructure and intensify the intention of the Naturopathic Reiki therapist and the open recipient.

Reiki Power Moves for Distance Healing

A Reiki power move using Hon sha ze sho nen is first spiritual in nature. Anything that you do with this symbol will be of a metaphysic nature. When using Hon sha ze sho nen, draw or visualize the symbol at the beginning of treatment, speak the name of your intended recipient and begin Reiki.

Hon sha ze sho nen establishes inner peace. Just like a prayer Hon sha ze sho nen stills the mind to accept empowerment to make changes in life.

Hon sha ze sho nen is used for connecting people. If your client has a need to join forces with someone for peace, progress or prosperity, Reiki can link the inner beings of the two people to encourage a physical connection.

Hon sha ze sho nen can also be used for disconnecting

people. When the client has past relationship problems that are still affecting them in the present and need courage or guidance on how to peacefully release the person, Hon sha ze sho nen can facilitate the merging of the two individuals where the immersion into oneness no longer causes an attachment issue.

Hon sha ze sho nen eases the mind of individuals that have issues with places from the past, present or future that cause anxiety. Places exist in our reality as markers for our experiences. Places also are linked to living purpose, as no one is ever in a place that they are not supposed to be, and often people who walk without this knowledge will have issues with places in time. Hon sha ze sho nen helps to bridge the gap to accepting that all places are steps in materializing the foundations needed to grow.

Hon sha ze sho nen can bring together ideas and ways of thinking that have existed for centuries. Often times solutions to problems are not in the present or future, instead they may be in the past. Hon sha ze sho nen can assist the individual with connecting ideas across dimensions of time and past life memories. Hon sha ze sho nen helps us to remember the minds of the ancients.

Hon sha ze sho nen can also ease anxieties about events in the future. Worry is giving to the mind more than what is necessary at the moment. When this occurs, the individual starts to formulate images and thoughts of things that could but have not happened and probably never will happen. Use Hon sha ze sho nen in Reiki therapy to settle the anxious thoughts of worry.

When a person has put up mental blocks that prevent them from moving forward in life or a situation, Hon sha ze sho nen corrects distortions that become obstacles to using the mind for the higher good.

Hon sha ze sho nen also helps seekers of higher spiritual clarity to bring a greater sense of enlightenment and spiritual awareness to a situation. Hon sha ze sho nen is also used to access divine will.

Distance is not a factor with Hon sha ze sho nen. Bring together the past, present and future into the healing circle of light.

Distance Healing

There are many ways to accomplish distance healing. Some therapists hold their hands up toward the person or group as pictured below. Most Naturopathic Reiki therapists find they can beam or send the remote treatment without raising their hands.

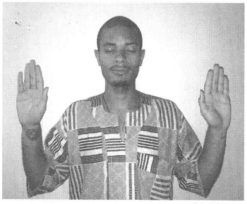

The following techniques have been used to send distant healing and are well established in the second degree of Naturopathic Reiki.

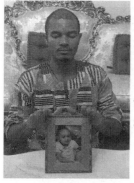

Draw the symbol over a photo of the recipient with the intention of sending Naturopathic Reiki.

Say the recipient's name while placing your hands in the distant healing hand position.

Direct the energies by imagining the person is resting in your lap.

Imagine the person in between your hands while you go through the hand treatment hand positions in your mind.

Send Reiki to the entire body of the intended recipient as one full body treatment.

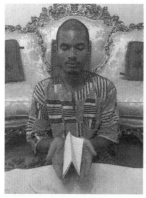

Write the person's name on a piece of paper and hold it between your hands and send Reiki.

Visualize the person there in the room with you and do the treatment.

Substitute your body for the recipient and intend that the energies run to them in the same places.

You can also spot treatment on a specific organ in the body. Just visualize it.

Ask your Reiki guides to undertake the treatment as you hold the connection.

State the condition that the treatment is for, if you know. Ask for pain relief, alleviate mental oppression, etc.

Distance treatment is suggested to run for fifteen to twenty minutes. The energy will run until it is done. Some have found that they get results from just five to ten minute sessions. End distance therapy by honoring what you have intended. Gently release the connection with an aura sweep.

***When you say Hon sha ze sho nen feel,
"the eternal omni presence."***

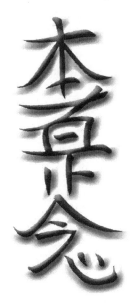

Hon sha ze sho nen Affirmations

- Right now. Hon sha ze sho nen.
- I am in the constant motion of timelessness, because I was before the first time and will be here beyond the last. I move today with the purpose of sharing the perfection that comes in living a life of truth. Hon sha ze sho nen.
- I free my soul from ignorance. I am not my body. I am the infinite peace of the universe. Hon sha ze sho nen.
- I devote myself to spiritual resurrection. Hon sha ze sho nen.
- I will remember the inspirations I have gained from the ancestors. Hon sha ze sho nen.
- I will roll with the light of the divine to the farthest reaches of the universe. Hon sha ze sho nen.
- I acknowledge that no relationship in this material world is actual; it is merely a reconnection of me to myself, a divine energy. Hon sha ze sho nen.

Hon sha ze sho nen Chants

The Hon sha ze sho nen chants call in the eternal presence of etheric energy and its ability to dissipate the illusion of separations and individualism. In Naturopathic Reiki to chant the mantras will align you as the Naturopathic Reiki therapist and your clients to the highest good of any situation or imbalance. Use these chants in private meditation time, during therapy, or as a personal exercise for your client to take with them and use for their own spiritual development.

- Hon sha ze sho nen is eternal.
- Hon sha ze sho nen brings me to balance.
- Hon sha ze sho nen is metaphysical truth.
- Hon sha ze sho nen is spiritual truth.
- Hon sha ze sho nen is divine.

The Hon sha ze sho nen Empowerment Plan

In addition to the 7 Days work in Cho ku rei and 7 Days with Sei he ki, there is also a 7 Day Empowerment Plan for Hon sha ze sho nen to help you get acquainted with using this symbol for the great works that you will do in Naturopathic Reiki.

Day 1 – For morning or evening meditation center yourself with the Gassho breath. When you are relaxed and ready chant the mantra Hon sha ze sho nen one time while visualizing the symbol going into your brow chakra. Give yourself a short Reiki treatment to close out the meditation.

Day 2 – Repeat day 1. In your Naturopathic Reiki journal practice writing the symbol Hon sha ze sho nen ten times.

Day 3 – Repeat day 1. Journal about any areas in your life that you need to use the power of Hon sha ze sho nen.

Day 4 – Repeat day 1. Mentally draw Hon sha ze sho nen and begin to visualize perfection of the areas in life that you journaled about yesterday. Conclude the visualization with the words, "Hon sha ze sho nen brings me balance."

Day 5 - For morning or evening meditation center yourself with the Gassho breath. When you are relaxed and ready chant the mantra Hon sha ze sho nen ten times while visualizing the symbol encircling the earth and vibrating out infinitely to the universe as far as you can imagine it going. Give yourself at least a fifteen-minute Reiki treatment to close out the meditation.

Day 6 – For morning or evening meditation center yourself with the Gassho breath. When you are relaxed and ready chant the mantra Hon sha ze sho nen ten times while visualizing the symbol connecting historical time periods as far back as you are aware of, then connect these events to present events in the world and then see the symbol connecting to the future as you imagine it or hope it to be. Give yourself at least a fifteen-minute Reiki treatment to close out the meditation.

Day 7 – For morning or evening meditation center yourself with the Gassho breath. When you are relaxed and ready chant the mantra Hon sha ze sho nen ten times while visualizing the symbol hovering in front of your brow chakra. When this focus is clear begin to chant, "no past, no present, no future; we are one." When you feel relaxed and complete send Hon sha ze sho nen all around your body in a beautiful indigo light that covers you from head to toe. You and Hon sha ze sho nen are now complete.

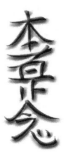

Additional Symbols

Ancient African in origin, **Ra** is an excellent symbol to add to Naturopathic Reiki. Ra represents solar energy that sustains all living things on earth. Ra is equivalent to Cho Ku Rei, universal power.

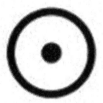

Ra Affirmations

- Every eye sees me on waking in the morning and my eye also sees every eye as well. Ra.
- The light that I am is eternal. As energy I am created in the form of truth. I live today in complete submission to who I am as the divine. Ra.
- My words are servants of my goodness. Ra.

The **ankh** is the Kemetic symbol of life and is used to encourage living life to the fullest. Its structure also reminds us of the interdependency we have for each other in the balance of masculine and feminine energy.

Ankh Affirmations

- I seek to internalize the laws of nature. Ankh.
- Everything I choose to consume will be natural. Ankh.
- I live in the realm of the spiritual masters. My body is my servant, its habits, addictions, cravings and desires have no control over my spiritual power. I, as spirit in physical form choose life. Ankh.
- Healing is the choice that moves me to magnificence. Ankh.
- I no longer fall to unrighteousness. I am purified. Ankh.

Chapter 3 Summary

The second degree of Naturopathic Reiki has three symbols that assist with understanding and applying the health care techniques involved in being a proficient Naturopathic Reiki therapist. Each symbol and mantra is designed to facilitate specific energy vibrations to raise the energy frequency of the recipient. Therapists are encouraged to use the symbols in both personal and professional care, beginning with the 7 Day Empowerment Plan for each symbol. Additional symbols can also be used based on the spiritual knowledge of the therapist.

*The affirmations used for all the symbols in this chapter can be found in the text _Today: Wellness Affirmations_ by K. Akua Gray.

Chapter 4

Naturopathic Reiki Therapy

Reiki therapies can be used for improving the physical health, easing the tensions of the mind, balancing the emotions and elevating the spiritual awareness of those who will receive this energy medicine. In this chapter, we will explore common therapies that have been used in Reiki with the symbols to assist with personal health and the health of clients.

Choosing the Right Music for Therapy

When a client first enters your professional space, they should feel the energy of healing immediately. One of the simplest ways of creating this atmosphere is through music. Music is a powerful energy vibration that is trance inducing, which is excellent for Naturopathic Reiki therapy. For the welcome, it is recommended to use music that encompasses the full range of musical notes throughout the composition, this stimulates the overall health and wellness of the client. Mellow African music and smooth jazz are examples of good welcoming music.

Once the initial assessment has been done and you have a good idea of what the client's needs are, this may call for a different kind of music. High vibrations in classical, flute and jazz music stimulate the mind and brain functions. When a client needs nurturing with relationships, memory communication, social skills, self-awareness, and emotional adjustments, high tones directly stimulate neurological functions. High tones also nurture the intuition, spiritual development, the brain's glandular functions and the ability to speak with openness and honesty. This type of music is excellent for the throat, brow and crown chakras.

Middle range tones affect the midsections of the body; the heart, lungs, stomach and all thoracic region organs are stimulated by soul, reggae, nature meditation, and pop music. This type of music is excellent for the heart and solar plexus chakras.

The lower tones stimulate the legs, knees, feet, and the reproductive system. Music with significant bass such as indigenous drums and rap music without the lyrics are excellent for intense stimulation. This type of music is excellent for the sacral and root chakras.

The music choice should always be in alignment with what the client needs to enhance the energy medicine experience. Keep the music volume low and comfortable for listening and organic conversation should the client want to communicate during therapy.

Reiki Meditation

Meditation is creating trance. Trance helps to release blocks and inhibitions for the recipient to receive the maximum benefit of the Naturopathic Reiki therapy. A brief meditation at the beginning of therapy is always a plus for both the therapist and the recipient. As a new Naturopathic Reiki therapist, there are two simple components to use that are sure to solidify the focus of the therapy: guided breathing and a brief affirmation. Depending on the client you may also use a guided visualization if the person is familiar with this type of mental stimulation.

The Four Count Breath brings complete focus to the third eye center with the ability to remove all thoughts from the mind. This powerful breath is used to affect the subconscious level of mind through the recitation

70

of affirmations during the breath work. This breath also stimulates the conscious mind's ability to affect the physical reality of a person.

Explain to your client that to start the Naturopathic Reiki session, you all will be doing a few minutes of guided breathing and affirmations. Have your client take a few deep breaths, and then have them to breathe along with your four-count finger snap or verbal count with each inhale and exhale. Repeat for four cycles and begin the affirmations. The affirmations are said by you, the therapist, while your client continues the rhythmic breath. After about four repetitions, slowly and quietly slow the affirmation to a close and begin the therapy.

If a visualization is to be used with a more spiritually advanced client, begin the visualization once the breath has been established. Visualizations should be no more than five minutes.

Reiki Symbol Treatment Programs

Self-Treatment for Emotional Healing
It has been mentioned before, as a Naturopathic Reiki therapist, you can only give what you have. If you are physically healthy and strong, then you can share your story of how you achieved good health. If you are mentally sound, you know the work that it took to reverse negative behaviors and retrain the way you think to reflect your divinity. If you are emotionally balanced, you can coach others to that emotional place of peace. If you are spiritually mature, you exude an air of grace and light that cannot be ignored and you can also share the self-journey to spiritual soundness.

On the other hand, if you are still working your way through these levels of ascension, that's ok too. Here is a very simple technique using Cho ku rei and Sei he ki that can bring ease to anything you may be going through in life.

Place your non-dominant hand at the base of your skull, upon the back of your neck, then with your dominant hand over the top of your head draw the power symbol once while saying Cho ku rei three times, draw the emotional healing symbol Sei he ki once while saying the mantra three times, then draw the power symbol, again saying Cho ku rei three times. Now place your non-dominant hand over the crown as well . With both hands on the head, repeat your selected affirmation for 3 – 5 minutes. For example: "I now have what I need to move forward in my life in a new direction that leads me to my purpose. I have the wisdom, strength, courage, and love to follow through with what is for me." Make sure that whatever affirmation you use that all of your words are positive and in the present tense.

The Emotional Healing Program
Reiki cannot erase the memory, nor should it, but removing the pain relieves the individual of the burden of the experience and they can then move on with their lives (Glaser 2016)

The Emotional Healing Program is accomplished in three phases that are essential in healing emotional blocks that have manifested as physical ailments and chronic conditions. The components of infusion, visualization, and affirmations are designed to bring to the surface and release negative conditions. The emotional program may be implemented before regular Reiki treatments. However, as a precaution if you are to do this program with a client, it is recommended to get a sound commitment from the client that they will complete the entire program. This program may seem small or innocent, but it can have severely detrimental and far-reaching negative consequences if it is not done properly. The program cannot be reversed because the visualizations are vivid reminders of traumas or unpleasant things a client has experienced, such as molestation, rape or a traumatic accident. It is also important to note that very personal information may be revealed with this treatment, therefore your commitment to client confidentiality is non-compromising. What happens in this therapy stays in this therapy.

Phase I – The Infusion

- Have the client to lie down and regulate their breath to a meditative state.
- When this is achieved, have the client to connect to the issue by visualizing themselves going through the ordeal all over again.
- Draw Hon sha ze sho nen and see it going into the client's crown chakra.
- Draw Cho ku rei and see it going into the client's crown, third eye, and heart chakra.
- Draw the Sei he ki and see it going into each chakra from the base to the crown.
- Finally draw Cho ku rei and see it covering the client's entire body.

Phase II – Visualization Therapy

- Put your hands in the face or head position whichever way is most comfortable.
- See the client's head and body filling with golden light.
- When the body is filled and overflowing, from the feet guide the golden light outside the body and

loop it back around to the crown chakra seeing it flow continuously through each chakra in a constant loop. This is sending purifying energy to the client.

Phase III – Affirmations

+ When the visualization reaches the continuous flow of energy, begin the affirmation.
+ Speak these words out loud to your client. "I send light, (Name), to the divine inner you, bringing love to all your needs. You are whole and free.
+ Continue the affirmation for 15 - 30 minutes. At the conclusion of the affirmation, you can proceed with the regular Reiki treatment.
+ Do the program for 3 days in a row, then leave it for a month or so to watch for developments before doing it again.

This is a very powerful program. It has helped individuals and families heal wounds of the heart, mind and soul.

Releasing Emotional and Mental Blocks
The trials of living in this modern world can bring about various imbalances that sometimes just need a quick release to help us maintain balance. This simple technique can be used to release and remove blocked energy or negative feelings for yourself and your clients quickly. Hold your Reiki hands outward in front of the throat and heart, visualize Sei he ki, and state your intention to release the negative energy and allow Reiki to flow as usual.

Mental and Behavioral Healing

Reiki is not a substitute for psychotherapy, medical treatment, or professional counseling, however, Reiki is complimentary to physician lead healthcare programs. On a spiritual level, Reiki is valuable and protective, however, people with serious psychological conditions should receive therapy from a Reiki therapist that also have credentials in the appropriate fields. Please use caution with clients who have known psychological issues as unsafe challenges may arise. Reiki can be used affectively for these types of conditions, but do not analyze anyone unless you are qualified.

In mental healing, Reiki works by removing energy blocks from the mind by stimulating the glandular functions of the brain. People hold conditioning, the causes of problems, and the mental impact of illnesses in the conscious and subconscious minds. Therefore, encouraging your client to actively seek mental solutions is always helpful. Self-treatment for some is easier for mental healing than from a therapist.

A stumbling block in mental healing for many is their belief system, especially as it pertains to religion. People can resist mental healing if they really don't want it. This is common in addicts, in people with parental issues and due to societal programming. Mental healing may require multiple sessions; however, there are no guarantees of any specific outcomes. You cannot force healing of a mental issue. Do not try to direct a specific outcome.

People are very susceptible to suggestion. Affirmations that you and the client have chosen are very powerful for mental healing, however, be very careful about what you say.

Death and Bereavement
Death is a normal reality of life, however, most people live with a profound and real fear of death. Naturopathic Reiki is a tool for enlightenment and losing the fear of death is one of the benefits of gaining spiritual consciousness to live the cycle of life.

You may one day be asked to assist a client in helping them maintain their life in the face of illness or an accident, or the life of a loved one in a similar situation. A part of understanding how energy works is accepting that sometimes disease and confinement to hospice is intended by the creator to be the final experience in a person's life. It is not for us as Naturopathic Reiki therapists to decide anyone's journey.

People who are in terminal states sometimes receive healing and live beyond expectations. Naturopathic Reiki can help a person die with less pain and emotional turmoil. Naturopathic Reiki can also help people become aware of the reality of continuing existence after death because energy never dies, it only changes form and frequency. It is always helpful to explain this to a client or family member because often they may have unrealistic expectations of what Reiki can do. Naturopathic Reiki therapists do not perform miracles and never promise cures. Some people find that Reiki helps them to move on to death with comfort. Reiki can be used with the intention that it eases transition and that it brings solace to the bereaved. It can also help clients recognize issues they need to deal with prior to passing over. Naturopathic Reiki helps eliminate the fear and anger that people feel surrounding death. Most of all, it helps connect with divine energy and the awareness that death is transition and not the end.

High Frequency Reiki for Pain Relief
Pain is a signal from the body that stress, disease or an invader has interrupted normal function. When a client needs Naturopathic Reiki for pain relief, it is helpful to know the cause of the pain. Once the cause has been established, you are able to focus the therapy with Cho ku rei as the frequency booster to the conscious, sub conscious and unconscious factors behind the pain. If the person is stressed to the point of physical pain, concentrate Cho ku rei in the upper body hand positions. If the person is experiencing pain from disease, concentrate Cho ku rei in the physical systems of the body. If the person is suffering pain from an accident, a cut or wound, a sprain or strain, focus Cho ku rei in that specific area.

When Naturopathic Reiki is concentrated and boosted with Cho ku rei it raises the frequency of the energy creating an intense portal of cellular realignment. Most times the pain is instantly relieved.

Group Healing
It is a common tradition among indigenous societies for healing to be a community effort. It is with this spirit that we explore Naturopathic Reiki group healing commonly known as Reiki circles. Group healing is where two or more Reiki therapists come together to share the power of Reiki as a unified force. This method of therapy is used for chronic conditions, catastrophes, and unusual circumstances. Sometimes the skills of a Naturopathic Reiki master may be needed to assist the novice.

Reiki for Children
Reiki is an excellent therapy for children. When treating children, make the therapy short, five to fifteen

minutes. Reiki for children works best at bed time. Naturopathic Reiki can be used to ease common childhood aliments like fever, toothache, eczema, rashes and bruises. However, be reminded that Reiki is not a substitute for medical treatment when needed. Ankh is a very good symbol to use with children.

Reiki for the Material State

Cho ku rei can be used to change the energy frequency of inanimate objects also. When an object is directly involved in the emotional and mental imbalance of a person, Reiki can dissipate energy debris from around the object that may be affecting the person.

Reiki for Pets

All living things can benefit from Reiki. Pets are sources of energy vibrations in our lives. People love their pets and want them to be healthy and live long. Like children the therapy that is given to domesticated pets should be short. It is not advisable to touch wild animals. Therapy in these cases should be distance healing with Hon sha ze sho nen.

Distance Healing for Energy Blocks

Hon sha ze sho nen in Reiki therapy is also done in the presence of the client to remove stress, trauma, and repression. These episodes create blocks, overloads, and scars that prevent healthy living. If these ailments are not healed, they can manifest as disease, mental illness, depression, anger and more. These issues can also cause antisocial and unpleasant behaviors. What some people don't realize is that these issues, especially if they become chronic, may be blocks from a past life. Distance healing would be helpful in these cases.

Distant Group Treatments
Reiki can be sent to more than one person or a group of
people all at once. As the Naturopathic Reiki therapist,
you are a conduit for the universal energy which
knows no space and time. This method can be used for
conferences, international conflicts, government bodies, or any small or large group gathering. Use what is
referred to as the *Blanket Method.* Visualize Cho ku rei,
Sei he ki and Hon sha ze sho nen collectively or individ-
ually, depending on the need, horizontally expanding
over the group of people or the area to be covered.
Adding a mental image of fanning the energy out over
the area or the people will help you focus.

Chapter 4 Summary

Naturopathic Reiki second degree therapies are intended for the beginning therapist to explore additional
ways of serving with the universal life force. The therapies are a variety of ways to get acquainted with using
the Reiki symbols with clients. There are also a variety
of ways to administer Reiki to other members of the
community including children, animals and inanimate
objects.

To master these therapies gives the therapist a solid
foundation to ready themselves for the third degree of
Naturopathic Reiki and its expansive repertoire of
higher spiritual modalities.

Chapter 5

Reiki Crystal Therapy

Crystal therapy is a great compliment to Naturopathic Reiki therapy. The sublunary properties of the richness of the earth come to life when crystals and stones are honored for their healing capabilities. Crystals and gemstones have been used in ancient times as far back as the first civilizations and dynasties in Africa. Today the practice of using stones and crystals continues. Crystal therapists know that the stones work as conductors to focus energy via a person's thoughts and chakras to stimulate healing both the physical and non-physical. Crystals are used in meditation and spiritual ceremonies, massage, bodywork, for relaxation, bathing, and other healing modalities. Using certain crystal methods can help a number of physical problems.

A crystal is composed of molecules that are organized and arranged in a consistent energy pattern. Crystalline molecules are naturally coordinated, synchronized, and balanced with one another. They are a reflection of a unified energy field and share a harmonic vibration with universal energy. The vibration from a crystal connects individuals in its presence with one pulsating energy wave.

Before you connect with a crystal of your choice, it should be cleaned to remove any unwanted energy that may have attached itself to the crystal prior to it coming into your life. Try one of these cleansing techniques as any one of them will do the job. Set your crystal in the sun for several hours, soak it in sea salted water overnight, bury it in the ground overnight, or smudge it with your preferred smudging method.

There are three types of crystals in the second degree of Naturopathic Reiki that work well with the three symbols. Clear quartz, calcite and amethyst form an alliance with the symbols to enhance the power of Reiki through physical representations of universal energy.

Clear Quartz
Clear quartz is the most diverse crystal to use in Reiki therapy. The versatility of clear quartz is found not only in its energizing effects, but also the shape of the crystal generates specific energies that aligns it perfectly with Cho ku rei. In general, clear quartz is used to cleanse, energize, open mental channels for insights, calm the emotions and heighten spiritual awareness. Literally, it can be used in Naturopathic Reiki therapy for everything. Like Cho ku rei, clear quartz vibrates with an elevated frequency that leaves no room for interference from low vibrations. Also clear quartz can be used for unblocking and balancing all chakras.

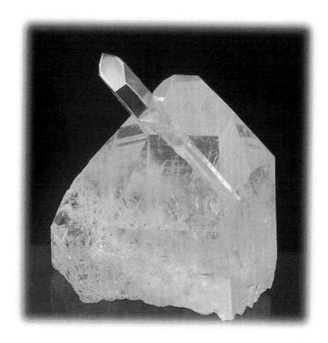

Some specific uses for clear quartz include:
- Settling family disputes
- Creating harmony in groups
- Spiritual insights for family problems
- In meditation to open chakras
- In meditation to assist with community problems
- Remove self-limitations
- Dissipate energy blockages
- Activate internal growth
- Stimulate the intellect
- Promote healing in the subtle bodies
- Charge spaces with positive energy
- Store, amplify and transmit spiritual energy
- Helps the individual to face their challenges
- Restores joy and hope
- Helps to heal childhood issues that are blocking growth
- Heightens all spiritual work
- Increases metaphysical intuition
- Improves communication

To expand your knowledge on clear quartz including the differences in the shapes and how it specializes the power of the frequency, research the following:
- Barnacle Crystal
- Bridge Crystal
- Double Terminated Crystal
- Faden-Lined Crystal
- Gemini Crystal
- Generator Crystal
- Growth Interference Crystal
- Isis Crystal
- Rainbow Crystal
- Tabular Crystal

Clear quartz basic body configurations in therapy are a great start for your crystal therapy work with yourself and your clients.

Core Infusion
Crystal on the hara.
This infusion strengthens the physical body.

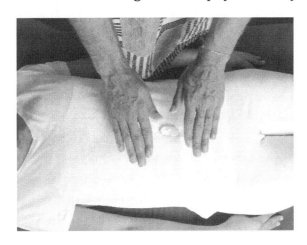

Full Body Grid
Create a diamond shape.
This grid assists with rebuilding the aura.

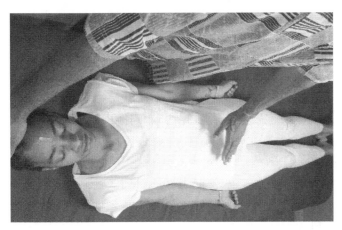

Chakra Boost
Crystals on each major chakra.

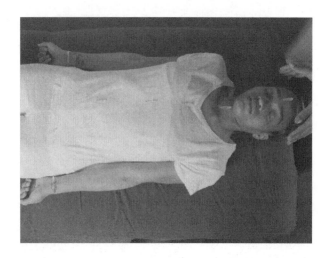

Personal Charge
Place a crystal in each hand of the recipient.

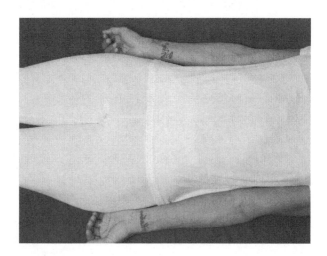

Calcite
Calcite is the go to crystal for all issues where Sei he ki is necessary in therapy. Calcite comes in various colors with orange, green and blue being the most popular. True to its name, calcite is known for its high calcium content which is a component in all soils around the world. Thus, every living thing needs calcium. Calcite works on elevating matters of a sublunary nature to the frequency of the heart vibration. It is not in the nature of calcite to induce spiritual ascension, therefore, it is most effective in root and sacral chakra work.

Calcite can be used to assist the body with nutrient absorption, making it excellent for bone and joint issues. It cleanses the emotions. Wherever emotional stress exist, calcite has a binding energy that directly affects the limbic system with a grounding effect. Therefore, use calcite for all emotional upheavals and imbalances.

Use calcite for the following basic body emotional energy release positions in therapy.

Abandonment
Place green calcite at the heart chakra.

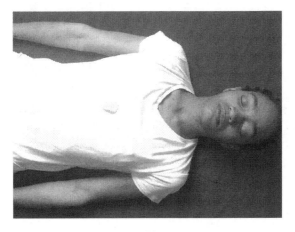

Anger
Place blue calcite over the liver.

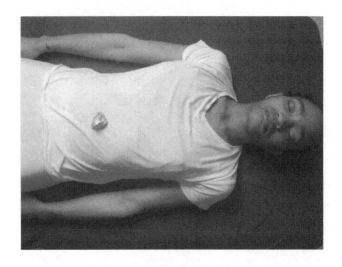

Bitterness
Place yellow calcite at the solar plexus.

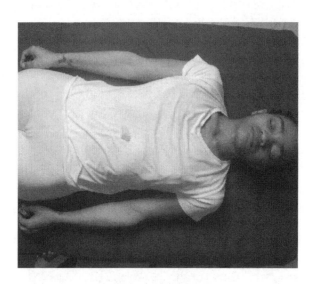

Fear
Place blue calcite on the left and right sides at the
kidneys.

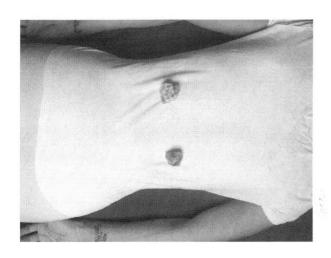

Guilt
Place orange calcite at the sacral chakra.

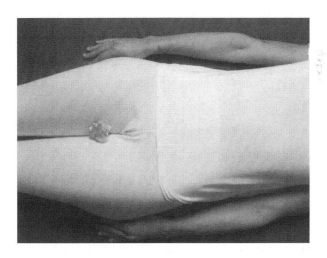

Sadness
Place green calcite just underneath the left breast.

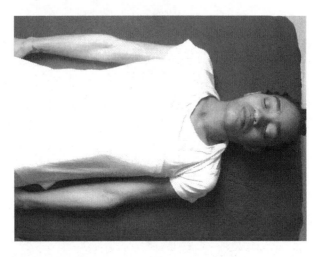

Amethyst
Amethyst is a curing crystal that opens the crown chakra. Amethyst radiates at the highest frequency level in the crystal family. Its Reiki symbol equivalent is Hon sha ze sho nen because amethyst works as a spiritual tuner that gathers information from the unconscious realm and formulates a channel of energy to the conscious realm making it a conduit for connecting places, people and energies over multidimensional space and time.

Amethyst facilitates a high vibration most people cannot absorb, therefore, it is recommended to only use this crystal in the upper chakras when the nature of the spiritual work is fully understood by the recipient and they are inviting the blessings of change with an open spirit. The energy in amethyst helps to boost the nervous system, increase the energy frequencies of the neurons in the brain, enhance the function of the pineal gland, and induces trance for greater reception.

Use these amethyst basic body configurations to increase the spiritual energy flow in therapy.

The Energy Ray
Place amethyst at the center of the top of the head.
This is a super stimulator for the brain and spine.

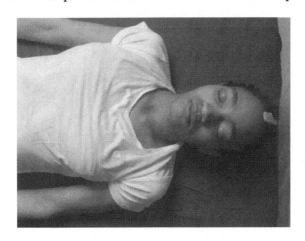

The Lotus Bloom
Place seven amethyst crystals from ear to ear over the head. This grid opens the entire etheric system for multidimensional subliminal communication.

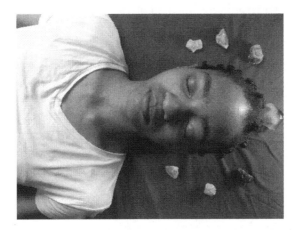

The Divining Rod
Place amethyst on the crown, brow and throat chakras.
This grid opens all clairvoyant channels.

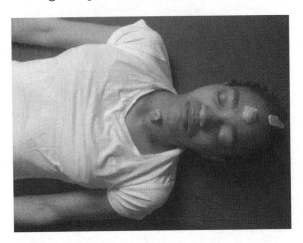

Crystal Tools and Techniques

Two very meaningful techniques with crystals that are used by many Reiki therapists include pendulum and wand work. Both these tools are readily available for purchase online, in many esoteric shops and at health food stores. Crystal tools help with focusing, reading energy, empowering, and cleansing. To become proficient in Naturopathic Reiki therapy takes practice. You are encouraged to choose crystals that "speak to your spirit" and have the qualities that are in alignment with your mission for providing good health care.

The Pendulum
Working with the pendulum in the second degree of Naturopathic Reiki is focused on the chakras. It is used to determine the viability of the recipient's energy centers. The pendulum will help you to determine which chakras are blocked, congested or free flowing. Clients always find this interesting to know what chakras are

clogged, and most will confirm and make commitments to personally work on those areas of their lives.

Preparing for Pendulum Chakra Reading
- ◆ Choose a pendulum that you are attracted to.
- ◆ Cleanse your pendulum by soaking it in salt water overnight.
- ◆ Program your pendulum by speaking your words of intention and setting your patterns of movement. (*Demonstrated in the Naturopathic Reiki II Certification course*).
- ◆ Once the patterns of movement are confirmed, your pendulum is ready.

Reading the chakras can be done in two ways, either as a part of your initial assessment with your client or as a therapist only assessment once your client is relaxed and ready for therapy. In the initial assessment, if you want to discuss with your client the health of their energy centers, you can use the sitting position hand assessment.

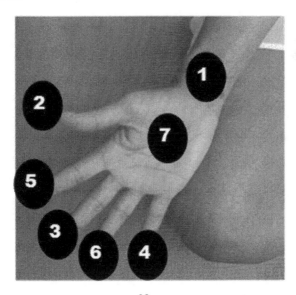

Have the client to hold out their dominant hand with fingers slightly spread. With a steady hand hold the pendulum over each noted area. The pendulum will respond based on the energy flow or lack thereof according to its programming.

1 Root Chakra - wrist
2 Sacral Chakra - thumb
3 Solar Plexus Chakra – middle finger
4 Heart Chakra – smallest finger
5 Throat Chakra – index finer
6 Brow Chakra – ring finger
7 Crown Chakra – center of the palm

For the therapist only assessment, the client is relaxed on the Reiki table with eyes closed. The therapist then uses the pendulum to assess the line of chakras along the governing vessel. Once the assessment is complete, the therapist can proceed to Reiki Chakra Therapy which we will discuss in the next chapter.

The Reiki Wand
The Reiki wand has also become a staple in tools used by Reiki therapists. Wands are made of various types of crystals, stones or gems, various shapes and sizes, and with various symbol engravings to suit the therapists' preferences. The wand has five distinct uses to enhance therapist ability and energy facilitation.

♦ Drawing the symbols
♦ Unblocking the chakras
♦ Cleansing the aura
♦ Charging the aura
♦ Channeling Reiki

The Reiki wand can be used to draw the Reiki symbols during therapy, which easily manifests the energy of the crystals that have been used for making the wand. For example, a wand made with lapis lazuli radiates a crown chakra energy vibration, thus to use this in drawing the symbols will boost spiritual reception for the client in the manner the symbols are being used.

To unblock the chakras, the Reiki wand is held over the chakra and rotated in a counterclockwise or pulsing motion to stimulate movement of the energy.

The Reiki wand is also used in the aura sweep to cleanse the aura. After the aura is cleansed, it is also important to clean your wand before doing any further wand work. Instructions for cleansing your wand with Reiki is forthcoming in the next section.

The aura can be charged by encircling the entire body with the wand, balancing the energy at the cardinal and intermediate points and then giving one big sweep of Reiki up the body from the foot to the head.

The Reiki wand can also double as Reiki hands, channeling Reiki just as if you were using your hands. This method of channeling Reiki is used most often by the therapist that is well versed in the use of crystal therapy to affect the energy flow of the meridians.

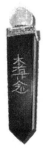 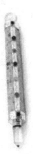

Clearing Your Crystals
It is good crystal therapy etiquette to clean the crystals you use in therapy after each client. Crystals gather energy from things and people they come in contact with. A very simple method is to place your crystals in a liter of water with a handful of sea salt. At minimum, allow them to soak for fifteen minutes.

Naturopathic Reiki II Aura Therapy and Cleansing

The aura is an energy force field around the body. It helps to protect, nurture and strengthen the inner and outer bodies of a person. When sickness occurs, there is a serious auric deficiency. This means the person's aura was not strong enough to repel the cause of the illness. The body's internal and external energy channels is a part of the built in medicine maker. Any type of imbalance is of a low vibration and the only way for lower vibrations to affect the body is if there is a compatible low or lower vibration to attach to. When the aura is energized and strong it is a natural repellent for disease.

Aura therapy as a method of prevention and to combat disease can be used with every advanced treatment of Reiki. Not only does it fortify the energy body, it boosts the immune system and rebuilds the protective energy matter that makes up the aura.

Method #1 Color Infusion
The color for infusing healing energy into the aura is green. When green shows up in a person's aura it radiates from the nutritive portion of the cells. This means that the body is balanced in hydration and nutrition. To infuse the aura with green light, channel Reiki to your heart and imagine a green ray coming from your heart

and covering the aura of your client. Hold this image for about five minutes, then run Reiki through the digestive system to enhance its function.

Method #2 The Reiki Symbol Method
Using the Reiki symbols in the aura is a normal occurrence for the professional Reiki therapist. The aura has been found to respond well when using the Reiki symbols. Cho ku rei is an automatic stimulator of the aura, use it when any of the chakras are blocked. Sei he ki increases the aura's illumination, use it when a client is dealing with darkness, sadness, depression and chronic fear. Hon sha ze sho nen creates an equilibrium between the inner and the outer auras. Use it when the client reveals an off and on lifestyle of health and wellness.

Method #3 The Ankh Method
Being that the ankh is the ancient symbol of life, this therapy is used to increase the energy of the client. When the client is suffering from fatigue or tiredness, begin Naturopathic Reiki therapy at the feet while picturing the ankh covering the body from head to toe. Then, proceed to the left side of the body placing the symbol into each area that Reiki is administered to. Next, apply therapy to the right side of the body with the same symbol infusion. The last position is at the crown, keeping the visual of the ankh covering the body from head to toe, begin to visualize the ankh rising from the person's body and lifting the aura up to a state of perfection. Your client should feel relaxed and energized after this treatment. A very effective addition to this therapy is to have a soft ankh chant playing in the background.

Method #4 Sweep and Energize

When the aura is found to be unhealthy, a very simple five-part method of sweeping the aura and energizing it with Naturopathic Reiki can restore auric protection. Starting on the left side of the body, sweep down the body from head to toe and touch the floor to release the stagnant energy. Then, sweep the inner left side of the body in the same manner. Next, sweep the right inner side of the body and finally sweep the outer right side of the body from head to toe, each time touching the floor to release the faulty energy. After the sweeping is complete, energize each chakra with three to five minutes of Reiki beginning from the first chakra to the seventh chakra and close the therapy with one final sweep and grounding down the center of the body.

Method #5 Strip and Release

This quick action method of cleansing the aura is widely used when there is not a lot of time for an extensive therapy. With hands spread wide and using a raking action, strip the aura from head to toe along the front of the body and touch the floor to release the stagnant energy. Do a few Gassho breaths to be sure you have maintained balance and standing at the client's feet release your hands up with a wave of Reiki energy back up the body and proceed with therapy or aura sweeping to close out the therapy.

Method #6 Breath Purification Technique

This guided aura therapy technique is done with the client's full participation. After a thorough reading of the chakras is complete and the aura is found to need reconditioning, have the client begin Mindful Breathing for about five minutes. When the breath is steady and a mild trance is induced direct the client to visualize with each inhale a powerful vibrant light of green energy coming into the lungs and with each exhale visualize the aura expanding inch by inch to its full luminance with every green breath. This visualization therapy last about ten minutes and will relax the client further to receive Reiki therapy.

Chapter 5 Summary

Naturopathic Reiki Crystal Therapy offers various high energy techniques to enhance the power and results of therapy for your clients. It is recommended to work with crystals that are relative to the power of the Reiki symbol as an introduction. The three recommended crystals are clear quartz with Cho ku rei, calcite with Sei he ki and amethyst with Ho sha ze sho nen.

Using crystal therapy tools focus and intensify the Reiki experience through energy readings and therapy with the crystal pendulum and the crystal Reiki wand.
The final aspect of crystal therapy to build on in your professional Naturopathic Reiki service is aura therapy and cleansing. Using the methods can strengthen the body's defenses to avoid sickness and repair the energetic power of the aura.

Chapter 6

Reiki Chakra Therapy

A Second Look at Chakras

Chakras can be explored and studied for decades by an individual and there would still be something new to learn about them in the end. In this second look at the chakras, it is intended to give the Naturopathic Reiki therapist a greater knowledge to invoke the health properties of the chakras that will assist with holistic healing. Holistic health returns the body, mind and spirit to nature to re-member what is most important to live a healthy life.

Root Chakra – Ankh

The root chakra internally gives energy to the function of the colon, kidneys, adrenals and spine. The body systems of this chakra are the digestive system, the excretory system, the muscular system and the nervous system. External physical properties include issues of strength and weaknesses of the feet and legs.

The natural intuitive sense of this chakra is the sense of smell, which is the guiding factor for other physical manifestations. Though many do not recognize their ability to identify with the scent of their natural surroundings, it is still an active part of the most primitive connection between people. Therefore, the minor chakra of the nasal passage is directly interrelated to the root chakra.

Balancing this chakra provides the physical body with the unlimited energy needed to increase overall health through the qualities of courage, patience and instinct.

Sacral Chakra – Khepera

The sacral chakra internally gives energy to the ovaries, womb, vagina, testicles, prostate, spleen and bladder. The body systems of this chakra are the reproductive system, the circulatory system and the excretory system. The external physical properties include issues concerning the penis.

The natural intuitive sense of the sacral chakra is the sense of (taste.) You can only taste what you smell, therefore, the interconnectedness of the first two chakras align the physical person with nature in its most primal relationship of survival and growth. There is a minor chakra on the tip of the tongue that causes a sensational physical movement of the tongue when the areas of the body that are governed by the sacral chakra are stimulated. This is the reason oral sex is a normal sexual act for mammals. In the third degree of Naturopathic Reiki, students are taught the appropriate hand position that correlates with applying Reiki to the tongue.

Balancing this chakra improves sexual vitality, physical power, fertility and creativity. It enhances the ability to master self-care, to give unconditionally, change without attachment and assimilate new ideas.

Solar Plexus Chakra – Ra
The solar plexus internally gives energy to the pancreas, stomach, liver, gall bladder, nerves and muscles. The body systems of the solar plexus are the digestive system, the muscular system and the nervous system. The external physical properties include the movement of the limbs.

The natural intuitive sense of the solar plexus chakra is the sense of (sight.) What we are able to see facilitates the structure for a physical relationship and the realization of all physical manifestations. Giving Reiki to the eyes helps the client to maintain a connection to the higher vibrations of physical existence. When a person can truly see without the illusions of society their life becomes their own. Giving Naturopathic Reiki through the eyes projects a higher level of Reiki energy that comes from the crown down through the solar plexus and back up through the eyes. This is why when a person is caught staring at someone the first place their eyes divert to is their abdomen to stave off the energy from its source.

Balancing this chakra strengthens the intuition, calms the emotions in three seconds or less, eases tension throughout the body and eliminates excessive frustrations.

Heart Chakra ~ Eye of Haku
The heart chakra internally works with the regulation of the heart, veins, arteries, lungs and thymus gland. The body systems of the heart chakra are the cardiovascular system, the limbic system, the respiratory system and the endocrine system. The external physical properties include the arms and hands.

The natural intuitive sense of the heart chakra is the sense of touch. Only after the sensual encounters of smell, taste and sight is a person open for the encounter of touch. The physical connection in touch assists with activating the higher senses. There are over 200 million touch sensors over the skin from head to toe. This makes the connection to the heart chakra easy through the integumentary system. Any time the body is touched, the vibrational sensation enters the heart both physically and spiritually. This is why touch in both negative and positive ways have been used to shape the behaviors of people. Negative forceful touch depletes energy and trains the mind and body to live in fear. Positive high vibration touch opens the heart, which stimulates the body to the sensations of living that helps a person to grow to their fullest potential. This is another reason why Naturopathic Reiki therapy is vital for mankind.

Balancing this chakra is important for the entire body. It increases the effects of spiritual love and universal oneness.

Throat Chakra – Ma'at
This chakra internally works through the auditory system and endocrine system, specifically with the thyroid, parathyroid, and hypothalamus. The external physical property is the mouth.

The natural intuitive sense is the sense of hearing. To hear at its highest level involves receiving sound vibrations externally and internally. With true hearing one is able to translate tone, frequency, force and inflection for the intended message. Many people find that their words and the words of others are the source of many miseries in life. There are minor chakras in the upper and lower lips that can be a point of focus in Reiki therapy when working with the throat chakra.

Balancing this chakra is important for speaking the truth, communicating with confidence and opening the communication areas of the brain as in telepathy.

Brow Chakra – Eye of Tehuti
The third eye chakra internally guides the pineal and pituitary glands through the endocrine system. The external physical properties include the left eye, nose and ears.

The natural intuitive sense of the third eye is the spiritual sense. Awareness of this sense is within the realms of the unseen. To access this sense for intention usually involves meditation for the novice or waking trance for the enlighten beings. Reiki therapy with the brow chakra and the aura go hand in hand.

Balancing this chakra enhances psychic perception, empowers the trust in one's intuition and promotes wise actions.

Crown Chakra *The Lotus*

The crown chakra internally aligns the pineal gland and cerebral cortex. The body systems governed by the crown chakra are the nervous system and the endocrine system. The external physical property is the right eye.

The natural intuitive sense of the crown chakra is the sense of enlightenment. Few seek to connect with this sense and even fewer achieve the task of connection. Use of this sense is achieved through many years of spiritual study, living and mastery of the sacred sciences.

Balancing this chakra creates bliss, vitality, and develops the psychic ability.

Energy Balancing Affirmations

Everything is energy vibration and can have a profoundly positive affect within the body. Affirmations can release emotions, tensions and stress. The words the body hears and feels from within is where powerful transformation starts. Each of the following can be used when working with organ regeneration, emotional balance, and relative situations in life.

Root Chakra
I know my divine self will fulfill all my needs.
My life is full and prosperous.

Sacral Chakra
I accept and acknowledge my sexual self.
My physical health is strong and pure.

Solar Plexus Chakra
In a calm and healthy way, I release my emotions.
I claim my personal power.

Heart Chakra
I freely give and receive love.
I totally forgive others and myself for all past errors.

Throat Chakra
I easily express my feelings and emotions.
I only speak words of truth.

Brow Chakra
My inner vision is clear and strong.
I trust my intuition and inner vision.

Crown Chakra
I accept and acknowledge my spirituality.
I am a god/goddess.

Elemental Chakra Therapy

Elemental Chakra Therapy is using the elements of air, fire, water, earth and spirit to enhance the chakra healing experience. Elemental Chakra Therapy can be applied in the form of minerals, plants, animals and people. The client indulges the senses with various aspects of the elements to release energy blockages. Presented here are a series of elemental chakra therapies and with consistent application can affectively change the overall alignment of the individual.

The Root Elements

The earth and its minerals offers a steady flow of healing energy to the root chakra. The primary place of being for all humankind is in the physical existence of the earth. The earth provides a constant magnetic draw to balance that most people ignore until they must come face to face with the repercussions of living an unnatural life.

The earth element during Naturopathic Reiki therapy is usually in the form of clay, stones or crystals.

The Sacral Elements

Water and its life-giving essence through the plant kingdom fuels the flow of the sacral chakra. Being 70% water and having the vital need of plant life for survival makes the connection to the procreation chakra understandable. Water nurtures and facilitates the basic movements of healing by the simple fact that we live on a water planet. The body is soothed by water. The spirit is moved by the sight of its grandness in the form of oceans, lakes, waterfalls, rivers, rain and snow. A return to elemental balance for the sacral chakra begins and ends with the Liquid Divine!

To eliminate the disconnect and the isolation methods of modern therapies, anytime a specific chakra is given a healing focus in Elemental Chakra Therapy, all chakras underneath must also receive attention in therapy. For example, the focus now is the sacral chakra, therefore the following therapy will include the root chakra element as well.

The water element during Naturopathic Reiki therapy is usually in the form of fountains, water sounds and a water based diffuser.

The Solar Plexus Elements
Fire and its ability to facilitate eternal change coupled with the animal kingdom's never ending story is the elemental highlight of the solar plexus chakra. If fire touches anything, it is never the same. Opening and balancing the solar plexus ignites the will to heal on all levels. The spirit stands at attention when fire is present, which renders it ready for action.

sun gazing

The fire element during Naturopathic Reiki therapy is usually in the form of candles.

The Heart Elements
Air as the element that sustains human motion is necessary at every moment of human life. The human kingdom cannot exist without the continuous facilitation of the energy of connection called love. Even those who live outside of their divine self unconsciously acknowledge that connection through their emotional responses to life and the outer body stimulus around them. The heart chakra vibrates unceasingly through the spirit of the air element, rippling the tones of eternity and change as a reminder to the human kingdom of who they are. Air. Energy. Vibration. One substance-divine.

The air element during Naturopathic Reiki therapy is usually in the form of breath work.

The Throat Elements
The ether realm of existence connects the human experience to the unseen. While the body exist in an illusion

of space and time, the unseen voice is the vehicle that expresses what the invisible mind chooses to share with the physical world. Speech comes forth only after the energy of mind allows the connection to the physical component of the body that brings forth sound. The voice and other elements of sound vibration have an exclusive power to transfix the mind in immediate suspension of time and space. When the voice is heard, there is an instantaneous magnetic draw to the ethereal realm from which the inner voice comes.

The ether realm or sound element during Naturopathic Reiki therapy is usually in the form of chants and affirmations. Chants should build, soothe, help, empower, create, relax and heal.
   ♀ My voice is my unseen power.
   ♀ My words become truth.
   ♀ I own my thoughts through my words.
   ♀ My voice is a force of healing.
   ♀ My words are peace.

The Brow Elements
The third eye element is spiritual vision. Having the ability to see and know what exist in the unseen world requires development of the brow chakra. The spirit world is the balance of the physical world, and as physical energy we take time naturally alternating between these worlds on a daily basis as our existence is primarily sensual. When one is able to intuit with precision and accuracy of the indwelling properties of life's daily engagements with the physical and spiritual realms, the third eye is open and the energy that empowers this portal fuels the physical actions of the person's life. Most people do not reach this level of awareness in their lifetimes. However, to give focus to this

area with the right tools will assist your client in developing ways of managing and maximizing those moments when the third eye is briefly activated in meditation and trance.

The visual element during Naturopathic Reiki therapy is meditation.

The Crown Elements
The crown chakra element is divine energy. It is a reconnection to source energy as the unconditional infinite supply of energy that is available for the use of everything in life. When an individual can tap into this energy the mind becomes vibrant with understanding and wisdom, the emotions become balanced and beneficial to all daily experiences, the physical body is nurtured to perfect health and longevity and the spiritual sense is always activated. Few people walk with this level of chakra activation. However, to give focus to this area with the right tools will assist your client in developing ways of managing and maximizing those moments when the crown is briefly activated in meditation and trance. Working with this chakra should include advanced breath work, an advanced level of meditation, the client should hold no fears of trance induction and they should be advanced in all lifestyle habits that promote wellness.

The divine energy element during Naturopathic Reiki therapy is usually in the form of advanced level meditation.

Chapter 6 Summary

Reiki and chakras is almost synonymous. It is the duality of the energy of healing that makes the study of chakras in Naturopathic Reiki vital. Reiki creates balance and chakras gauge that balance. Reiki Chakra Therapy is developing the advanced ability to assist clients with their physical, mental, emotional and spiritual health through specific hand positions, meditation, affirmations and chakra elemental therapy. Proficiency is achieved with regular therapy sessions.

Chapter 7

The Reiki Professional

Naturopathic Reiki therapy and every Naturopathic Reiki therapist is unique and fluid. Although Reiki has a solid foundation that is central to all well-trained therapists, the uniqueness of what you offer in professional style as you become proficient will be very different from how anyone else who provides Reiki as a holistic healthcare service. We have seen this evolution take place in more than twenty different types of Reiki over the past hundred years from Japan, Israel, Egypt, Tibet, India, Canada, The United Kingdom and The United States of America. Remember the uniqueness you bring to Naturopathic Reiki as a one of a kind therapist will be a part of the next one hundred years of world healing.

Setting Up Your Business
Providing a professional service in Naturopathic Reiki can be done in many ways. You can set up an independent office, have a mobile service, contract out to wellness centers, hospitals and doctor's offices or have a pop up service at wellness fairs. However you choose to set up your business, there are a few basic professional principles that are standard in holistic health service that should be applied with consistency for success. Run your business with integrity by clarifying your intention to facilitate and promote health and healing of the body, mind and spirit.

This starts with putting together a business plan that outlines your vision, your professional objective, your personal objective and information on the market you intend to serve. It's very easy to register your business with your local county or parish tax assessor's office. The documents you receive at registration will allow you to open your bank account(s) and reserves your business name in your local area usually for ten years.

After your business plan is in place and your registration is complete, you should then turn your attention to the service you are ready to provide. Every good business starts off with good marketing. A successful business maintains consistent marketing to the tune of three marketing efforts a day. There are numerous tools for marketing and it is suggested that you take marketing training for startup businesses if this will be your first endeavor or if marketing has not been a focus in your past businesses. The following are a few marketing tips to pick and choose from as you build your clientele.

* Set up a free website to start.
* Get business cards printed.
* Link up to your favorite social media and tell friends about your business.
* Attend a big community event to introduce your business to potential clients.
* Collaborate with others in the wellness field to tap into a wider audience.
* Develop repeat customer specials and multiple session packages.
* Have a referral special for clients who tell their family and friends about your business/services.

Just Like That

Now you are consistently getting the word out about your Naturopathic Reiki service. It's time to turn your focus to the professional therapy space that you have chosen. Always maintain a superior professional appearance. Wherever you provide your service, make sure it is a safe and comfortable environment. A healing space, even if it is out in public should have an air of relaxation.

Always remember you are in the service business, this means that you will set fees and be compensated for your time. Set your fees to reflect your market and your needs. Your time as a professional is valuable; know your worth. At present, Reiki standard fees have been in alignment with the massage therapy profession. Many therapists charge $1 to $2 per minute. If working at a spa or resort the command is three to five times as much, however, these high-end venues also add in very nice perks like juicing, a meal, a health assessment, and a complete day of relaxation.

Make your business unique and your originality will contribute greatly to your success.

Before Your Client Arrives
When preparing for your client make a checklist to refer to each time to ensure consistency in your delivery of service. Everything about your business environment should be neat, in order and clean. Your professional appearance and personal hygiene fits into this category too. Avoid heavy perfumes and heavily scented deodorants, remember your arm pits will be open with some hand positions. It is recommended to use the unscented version of your favorite natural deodorant.

Create and maintain a professional oath of confidentiality for all conversations, health information and session therapies for every client. All Naturopathic Reiki sessions are confidential including your client's mental and emotional state.

Before each client, take some time to prepare any forms that are needed for your records are on hand and ready to be completed. It is always a good idea to also provide a pen.

When preparing to receive your client, make sure the Reiki table is set with clean linen. Charge the therapy space with Reiki and do a mini treatment on yourself to ensure the open flow of your channel. Be relaxed, be enlivened and be Naturopathic Reiki ready!

When Your Client Arrives
Everything is ready. You greet them with a warm smile and begin to prepare them for treatment. Be honest with your clients. Establish rapport with full disclosure of what Naturopathic Reiki can and cannot do. It is standard to have a questions and answers moment before and after the therapy. Also, inform clients of the mechanics of Reiki therapy if they are not familiar with the techniques. Treat all clients with kindness and respect. Discrimination of any kind is unacceptable to this profession.

The Therapy Session
Wash your hands before and after the therapy. Each therapy session will be unique to each client. Please review Naturopathic Reiki Level I for a refresher on sharing Reiki and remember to explore your creativity in pattern and style of therapy. For example:
* Begin with guided breathing to relax the client.
* Scan the chakras to discover any blockages.
* Set crystals in place for a specific therapy.
* Do any cleansing techniques to remove any energetic debris that may cloud the therapy.
* Begin Naturopathic Reiki based on client needs or chakra reading.
* Treat the front and back of the body.
* Remove crystals to the salt water bowl.
* Do an aura sweep.
* Recheck the chakras.

115

* Quietly inform the client that the session has ended and give them plenty of time to come out of trance and ground themselves with a little drink of water.
* Also, give your client the opportunity to share their experience if desired and discuss their follow up appointment.

Have a referral system in place for clients who need assistance outside of your scope of service.

After Your Client Departs
Immediately clean your therapy space and personal aura to ensure you are detached from any energetic debris that may still be lingering. Take a few minutes to rest and enjoy the Reiki buzz that energizes you during every session. You should feel just as great as the client. It is a good idea to space your clients far enough apart to give yourself time to prepare for the next client and care for yourself in between therapies.

Update your client therapy log on the session and keep client records for up to three years.

Maintaining Your Positive Energy

When you choose the healing arts to share with the world, it requires a great deal of energy that counters the normal way people operate in everyday life. As a healer, there are some things that should change about you and how you conduct yourself among people. But to truly change the public you, you must change the private you first. You are encouraged to seek the ability to align life and purpose with the highest vibrations available to man.

The following are unacceptable behaviors in any wellness service. If any of these character or lifestyle habits are a part of the way you live, it is advisable that you work to change them before claiming to be a community healer:

* Eliminate violence, horror and negative news
* Eliminate using profanity and abusive language
* Eliminate urges or active solicitation of sex from your clients
* Eliminate using recreational drugs to get high
* Eliminate using alcohol for inebriation
* Eliminate arguing
* Eliminate living a self-defeating eating lifestyle
* Eliminate smoking anything that creates a carcinogen for the respiratory system
* Eliminate being a hypocrite in religion

If you need assistance with any of these changes, it is suggested to seek counseling, go through a spiritual rite of passage or study a higher level of spiritual development such as one of the Kemetic or other ancient spiritual systems.

Chapter 7 Summary

Becoming a great Naturopathic Reiki therapist doesn't take much time with consistency, however, growing a Naturopathic Reiki business can be a lengthy process. You are encouraged to start your business the right way in the beginning with proper business registration, market research, and providing a professional service that will speak for itself. Being a professional therapist starts before your clients arrive and continues after the day is done. Work hard and the love for what you do will pay off.

Chapter 8

Preparing to Become a
Naturopathic Reiki Master

Third degree Naturopathic Reiki is the master teacher level. It will prepare you to use the power of Reiki to its greatest capacity. There are few Reiki Masters compared to Reiki Level I Self-healers and Level II Professional therapists. Level three of Naturopathic Reiki is a great responsibility and requires a consistency in the use of Reiki to maintain the gift that the Master symbols offer. If you have a desire to expand your spiritual and mental ability to the super human level and teach others to do the same to continue to create a world where the energy of the creator is no longer a mystery, but an accessible norm for light workers, then, the third degree of Naturopathic Reiki could be for you.

Naturopathic Reiki II 90 Day Therapy Challenge

In Naturopathic Reiki Level I students completed a three-week clearing to get acclimated to both self-healing and sharing Naturopathic Reiki with others. In Naturopathic Reiki II for those who are interested in moving forward to Naturopathic Reiki Level III, the Master Teacher certification, we will embark upon a three-month journey to develop more spiritual awareness, develop originality in therapy and share Naturopathic Reiki with a minimum of fifty people.

Return to your Reiki vision board or journal and assess how much of your life has changed with the first degree of Naturopathic Reiki. Journal what areas you would like to continue to develop and use this as a guide for part one of the 90 Day Challenge of spiritual awareness.

Segment 1
For 90 days, maintain an active practice of meditation and positive declarations in your choice of spiritual

wisdom. Include 90 days of journaling to record your revelations and awareness.

Segment 2
Within the 90 days of spiritual awareness development you are required to give Naturopathic Reiki therapy to 50 people. This can be for paying clients or offered as a free service. Sessions must be at least 15 minutes and a journal log of each session should be recorded as validation of completing this aspect of the challenge.

Segment 3
Also, within the 90 days and the 50 sessions requirement, make a note in your journal of the unique therapy developments that come from this intensive practice. What new and interesting things have you added to your therapy that enhanced what you learned in Naturopathic Reiki II certification.

It would be great to share this with your Reiki Master teacher when you decide to move forward in receiving your Master attunement.

The Naturopathic Reiki Master Curriculum

Naturopathic Reiki III
To truly master a component of health care takes time. The Naturopathic Reiki III Master/Teacher Certification is an extensive training and a one year apprenticeship program. Students are required to complete an extensive study on spiritual healing that involve therapies, book studies and teaching assignments.

A Study on Spiritual Healing
Learn to hear, see and know what spirit can do in your life and the lives of your clients. Take a journey through the timeless teachings of Alan Young, the au-

thor of <u>Spiritual Healing: Miracle or Myth</u>.

Reading the Aura
The advance study of the aura involves developing the skills to see, feel and hear the energy that surrounds living things. Inside the aura is a world of understanding that is only available to the trained third eye.

The Symbols
The master symbols are universal vibrations of power that affect the cellular make up of living entities. Learn to use these powerful symbols and mantras to direct and enhance ki beyond the understanding to the normal mind.

Advanced Chakra Therapy
Everything in Naturopathic Reiki mastery is designed to remind the world that universal energy is the control mechanism for everything that happens in the physical world. Gain knowledge in the twelve major and forty-two minor chakras that are the real healing channels of the body.

Meridian Therapy
The meridians come to life in Naturopathic Reiki mastery as you learn to work with the meridians through scanning, cleansing and energizing techniques.

How Attunements Work
The highlight of Naturopathic Reiki mastery is learning the attunement process. Get lots of practice in this profound initiation process that brings immortality to Reiki as a healing channel.

Advanced Healing Techniques
This study in the <u>Complete Handbook of Dr. Usui Mikao</u> by Frank Ajaver Petter teaches one hundred year old therapy techniques that have been used around the world to bring balance to the health of millions.

Teaching Reiki
Teaching Reiki is a requirement for the one year apprenticeship in Naturopathic Reiki III. Learn how to conduct Reiki classes, develop curriculum and get hands on practical work in passing along the Reiki power to the novice who are also ready to carry light into the world.

The Master Path
The path is truly a journey that brings about permanent change. There is a legacy to uphold that encompasses the power of healers for more than a thousand generations. Be one of the legacy keepers by continuing to bring value and dignity to the work of the Reiki Master.

Recommended Naturopathic Reiki Master Preparations

* Successfully complete the Reiki II 90 Day work
* Make self-treatment a daily routine
* Read several Reiki books to become familiar with different styles and techniques
* Join or create a Reiki Circle in your community
* Stay in touch with your Reiki Master for guidance
* Join a Reiki network for support and updates
* Keep in touch with your Reiki classmates and share your experiences
* Strengthen everything about you on a mental, physical, emotional and spiritual level

The advanced levels of Naturopathic Reiki provide a channel into enlightenment. This has always been the intention of this healing art. Be ready to take on the responsibility that comes with great power.

Chapter 8 Summary

Preparing to become a Naturopathic Reiki Master is a serious decision. This knowledge opens doors to certain advantages that require responsible commitment to live righteously, to be able to give what is needed, to be a legacy builder for this ancient healing art. The curriculum and training is intensive. Take the time to adequately prepare for the journey by doing the work to prove to yourself that you are truly the one.

Recommended Reading List

Ra Sekhi Level Two
Rekhit Kajara Nebthet

Essential Reiki.
A Complete Guide to an Ancient Healing Art
Diane Stein

Modern Reiki Method for Healing
Hiroshi Doi

The Spirit of Reiki: From Tradition to the Present Fundamental Lines of Transmission, Original Writings, Mastery, Symbols, Treatments, Reiki as a ... in Life, and Much More (Shangri-La Series)
Walter Lubeck, Frank Arjava Petter
and William Lee Rand

Reiki Fire: New Information about the Origins of the Reiki Power: A Complete Manual (Shangri-La)
Walter Lubeck, Frank Arjava Petter
and William Lee Rand

Reiki Healer:
A Complete Guide to the Path and Practice of Reiki
Lawrence Ellyard

Reiki Energy Medicine: Bringing Healing Touch into Home, Hospital, and Hospice
Libby Barnett

Reiki & Medicine
Nancy Eos

Acknowledgements

Naturopathic Reiki is a system of Reiki that brings to focus the deeper effects on health that energy healing can have. People suffer unnecessarily and there is hope if this healing art is mastered by those who understand and live the principles of holistic health.

As a Reiki Master Teacher for more than a decade, I have worked with some outstanding students who have gone on to do great healing work in their community. Seeing their work has been an inspiration to ensure that there is a healer in every home. I send love and light to the two hundred and fifty-five students to date that I have trained in Reiki and I am grateful for you allowing me to share this peace knowledge with you so that you in turn can heal the world.

I also acknowledge the models, photographers, students, editors and designers who helped in bringing this ten year old manual to publishing. My number one photographer, supporter and love of my life-story Dr. Chenu Gray is the life line for great photos in all three volumes of the Naturopathic Reiki book series. My son, Kazembe Gray, especially made this Naturopathic Reiki II book a vibrant example of professional work with his eye for photography with models Chakory Dey and Nasira Mayfield. A special thank you to Naturopathic Doctor Bikeeyah Baht Ammi Kudiabor of Takoradi, Ghana for assisting with both Naturopathic Reiki I and Naturopathic Reiki II manuals. A special thank you also goes out to Fayola Herod "the editor" that I trust completely with her expertise and insight for the entire A Life Of Peace Wellness Therapy Series.

References

Amen, Ra Un Nefer (1990) Metu Neter Volume One: The Great Oracle of Tehuti and the Egyptian System of Spiritual Cultivation. New York, NY: Khamit Media Trans Visions Inc

Bridges, Faye. (2015) REIKI: Reiki Meditation: Strengthen Body & Spirit and Increase Energy with Reiki Healing and Meditation - Complete Guide Kindle Edition.

Corr, Kristine Marie (2015) Reiki: A Complete Guide to Real Reiki: How to Increase Vitality, Improve your Health and Feel Great. Maven Publishing. Kindle Edition.

Glaser, Angela (2016) Reiki Self-Healing 101: An Easy Introduction to Reiki Self-Healing. CreateSpace Independent Publishing Platform. Kindle Edition.

Gray, K. Akua (2016) Natural Health and Wellness: The Consultant Manual Missouri City, TX: BJK Publishing.

Morello, Tai. (2015) CHAKRAS: Chakras for Beginners: The Ultimate Guide to balance Your Chakras, Radiate Energy and Heal yourself. Kindle Edition.

Parnell, Chris and Ginger (2007) Reiki Manuals 1, 2 and 3 Spring, TX: Spirit Quest, LLC.

Petter, Frank Arjava (1999) The Original Reiki Handbook of Dr Mikao Usui. New Dehli, India: Lotus Press.

Pookrum, Jewel (1999) Vitamins and Minerals from A to Z. A&B Publishers Group: Brooklyn, NY

Quest, Penelope (2010) Reiki for Life: The Complete Guide to Reiki Practice for Levels 1, 2 & 3. New York, NY: TarcherPerigee.

Stevens, John O. (1988) Awareness: exploring experimenting experiencing. Eden Groves Edition: Great Britain

Yamashita, Alexander (2014) Reiki For Beginners: Master the Ancient Art of Reiki to Heal Yourself And Increase Your Energy. Kindle Edition.

Powerpoint Class Notes 10.04.20
Chapter 1 pg 8-10
"Knowledge of the Unseen" - Reiki

Where are You (self) vibrating?
- Low → > 300
- Normal → 300-400
- Reiki → 400-800
- Spiritual Master → < 800

A sound therapist has tuning forks to inform you as to where you are vibrating at (Hz)

counter clockwise = unblock cleansing

clockwise = energizing/restoring energy

Made in the USA
San Bernardino, CA
13 July 2020